FIELD GUIDE

to

OCCUPATIONAL THERAPY

for

PHYSICAL DYSFUNCTION

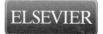

3251 Riverport Lane
St. Louis, Missouri 63043

MOSBY'S FIELD GUIDE TO OCCUPATIONAL THERAPY
FOR PHYSICAL DYSFUNCTION   ISBN: 978-0-323-06767-6

Notices

Knowledge and best practice in this field are constantly changing. As new research and experience broaden our understanding, changes in research methods, professional practices, or medical treatment may become necessary.

Practitioners and researchers must always rely on their own experience and knowledge in evaluating and using any information, methods, compounds, or experiments described herein. In using such information or methods they should be mindful of their own safety and the safety of others, including parties for whom they have a professional responsibility.

With respect to any drug or pharmaceutical products identified, readers are advised to check the most current information provided (i) on procedures featured or (ii) by the manufacturer of each product to be administered, to verify the recommended dose or formula, the method and duration of administration, and contraindications. It is the responsibility of practitioners, relying on their own experience and knowledge of their patients, to make diagnoses, to determine dosages and the best treatment for each individual patient, and to take all appropriate safety precautions.

To the fullest extent of the law, neither the Publisher nor the authors, contributors, or editors, assume any liability for any injury and/or damage to persons or property as a matter of products liability, negligence or otherwise, or from any use or operation of any methods, products, instructions, or ideas contained in the material herein.

ISBN: 978-0-323-06767-6

Vice President and Publisher: Linda Duncan
Executive Content Strategist: Kathy Falk
Content Manager: Jolynn Gower
Publishing Services Manager: Julie Eddy
Project Manager: Marquita Parker
Design Direction: Maggie Reid

Printed in the Unites States

Last digit is the print number: 9 8 7 6 5 4 3 2 1

Working together to grow
libraries in developing countries

www.elsevier.com | www.bookaid.org | www.sabre.org

ELSEVIER   BOOK AID International   Sabre Foundation

Expert Consultants

Cynthia Cooper, MFA, MA, OTR/L, CHT
Clinical Specialist in Hand Therapy
Faculty, Physical Therapy Orthopedic Residency Program
Scottsdale Healthcare
Scottsdale, Arizona

Lisa Deshaies, OTR/L, CHT
Adjunct Instructor of Clinical Occupational Therapy
Department of Occupational Science and Occupational Therapy
University of Southern California
Los Angeles, California
Occupational Therapy Clinical Specialist
Occupational Therapy Department
Rancho Los Amigos National Rehabilitation Center
Downey, California

Introduction

As a busy therapist or student in the clinic, having information at your fingertips is important. This field guide gives you quick reference to information commonly needed in practice—providing information on anatomy, assessment tools, screening tools, and much more in a quick-reference format to use for assessment and application, documentation, client education, or communication with clients and other health care professionals.

Mosby's Field Guide to Occupational Therapy for Physical Dysfunction is a unique handheld reference designed to assist the OT student and clinician, regardless of level of experience, with the basics of point-of-care assessment and treatment. On a daily basis, therapists need information on anatomy and physiology, precautions, applications, assessment pathology and pain, as well as record-keeping. Rather than flip through numerous large texts between clients, this book consolidates key information into one convenient, well-organized, portable guide for fast and easy lookup. The material in this field guide is compiled from *Pedretti's Occupational Therapy, 7E* and other resources in occupational therapy and other health care disciplines.

Mosby's Field Guide to Occupational Therapy for Physical Dysfunction will serve as the much-needed resource for students to guide them during clinical course work, for new therapists entering practice, and to occupational therapy assistant (OTA) programs because students in these programs must also be able to demonstrate competencies related to their basic practice skills.

Contents

Overview and Occupational Therapy Process

The Occupational Therapy Practice Framework and the Practice of Occupational Therapy for People with Physical Disabilities

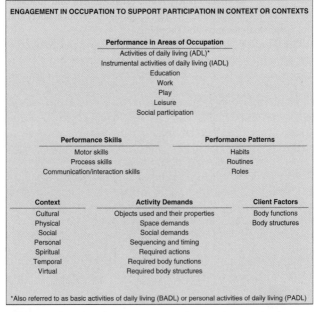

ENGAGEMENT IN OCCUPATION TO SUPPORT PARTICIPATION IN CONTEXT OR CONTEXTS

Performance in Areas of Occupation

Activities of daily living (ADL)*
Instrumental activities of daily living (IADL)
Education
Work
Play
Leisure
Social participation

Performance Skills	Performance Patterns
Motor skills	Habits
Process skills	Routines
Communication/interaction skills	Roles

Context	Activity Demands	Client Factors
Cultural	Objects used and their properties	Body functions
Physical	Space demands	Body structures
Social	Social demands	
Personal	Sequencing and timing	
Spiritual	Required actions	
Temporal	Required body functions	
Virtual	Required body structures	

*Also referred to as basic activities of daily living (BADL) or personal activities of daily living (PADL)

FIGURE 1-1 The six broad areas or categories of concern that comprise the occupational therapy domain include performance in areas of occupation, performance skills, performance patterns, context, activity demands, and client factors.

Activities of daily living (ADLs), also referred to as personal activities of daily living (PADLs) or basic activities of daily living (BADLs), are those activities that have to do with accomplishing one's own personal body care. The body care activities included in this category are bathing and showering, bowel and bladder management, dressing, eating, feeding, functional mobility, personal device care, personal hygiene and grooming, sexual activity, and toilet hygiene.

Instrumental activities of daily living (IADLs) are those activities that support daily life in the home and community and that often require more complex interactions than self-care used in ADLs. The specific IADLs include care of others (including selecting and supervising caregivers), care of pets, child rearing, communication management, community mobility, financial management, health management and maintenance, home establishment and management, meal preparation and cleanup, religious observance, safety and emergency maintenance, and shopping.

Rest and sleep includes activities related to obtaining restorative rest and sleep that supports healthy active engagement in other areas of occupation. The component activities comprising rest and sleep include rest, sleep, sleep preparation, and sleep participation.

Education includes activities needed for learning and participating in the environment. Specific education activity subcategories include formal education participation, informal personal educational needs or interests exploration (beyond formal education), and informal personal education participation.

Work includes activities associated with paid work and volunteer efforts. Specific categories of activities and concerns related to work include employment interests and pursuits, employment seeking and acquisition, job performance, retirement preparation and adjustment, volunteer exploration, and volunteer participation.

Activities associated with play are described as any spontaneous or organized activity that provides enjoyment, entertainment, amusement, or diversion. Considered under this area of occupation are play exploration and play participation.

Leisure is defined as nonobligatory activity that is intrinsically motivated and engaged in during discretionary time—that is, time not committed to obligatory occupations such as work, self-care, or sleep. Leisure exploration and leisure participation are the major categories of activity in the leisure area of occupation.

Social participation encompasses the organized patterns of behavior that are characteristic and expected of an individual or a given position within a social system. The area of social participation further encompasses engaging in activities that result in successful interaction at the community, family, and peer-friend levels.

The primary focus of *Occupational Therapy Practice Framework: Domain and Process,* 2nd edition (OTPF-2) is the evaluation of the client's occupational abilities and needs to determine and provide services (intervention) that foster and support occupational performance (outcomes). Throughout the process, the focus is on occupation; the evaluation begins with determining the client's occupational profile and occupational history. Preferred intervention methods are occupation-based and the overall outcome of the process is the client's health and participation in life through engagement in occupation (Fig. 1-2).

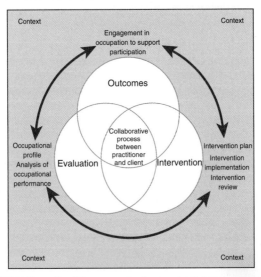

FIGURE 1-2 Occupational therapy practice framework collaborative process model.

BOX 1-1 Occupational Therapy Practice Framework: Quick Guide*

The framework is comprised of two interrelated parts: domain and process.

Domain
This is what OTs do; no single aspect is considered more critical than another.
    Performance in areas of occupation: ADLs, IADLs, rest and sleep, education, work, play, leisure, social participation
    Client factors: values, beliefs, and spirituality, body functions, body structures
    Activity demands: space demands, social demands, sequencing and timing, required actions, required body functions, required body structures
    Performance skills: motor and praxis, sensory perceptual skills, emotional regulation skills, cognitive skills, communication and social skills
    Performance patterns: habits, routines, roles, rituals
    Context and environment: cultural, personal, temporal, virtual, physical, social

BOX 1-1 Occupational Therapy Practice Framework:
Quick Guide—cont'd

Process

This is how OTs provide their services. It is a collaborative process between the client and OT.

Evaluation: occupational profile, analysis of occupational performance

Intervention: preferred term over *treatment*; includes intervention plan, intervention implementation, intervention review

Outcomes: all goals aimed at overarching goal of supporting health and participation in life through engagement in occupation

Client: recipient of OT services; preferred term, but actual term varies by practice setting; could be patient, student, consumer, employee, employer

Individual: broad view of client; could be actual person with a disability or individual providing support for the client, such as family, caregiver, teacher, employer, who also may help or be served indirectly

Organization: such as businesses, industries, agencies

Populations: within a community

Client-centered approach: an approach to the evaluation and provision of the intervention with emphasis on the client and his or her goals

Occupation versus activity: activities characterized as being meaningful and goal-directed but not of central importance to the life of the individual, whereas occupations are viewed as activities that give meaning to the person's life, contribute to one's identity, and are those in which the individual looks forward to engaging. In the OTPF-2, the term *occupation* encompasses activities.

Engagement: includes both the subjective emotional or psychological and objective physically observable aspects of performance.

Types of Intervention

Therapeutic use of self: OT uses own self and all that entails (knowledge, personality, experience), conveying empathy, active listening, establishing trust

Therapeutic use of occupations and activities

Occupation-based activity: client engages in the occupation

Purposeful activity: client learns and practices parts or portions of occupations.

Preparatory methods: methods that prepare client for purposeful or occupation-based activity

Consultation process: OT uses knowledge and expertise collaborating with client to identify problem, develop, and try solutions; up to client to implement final recommendation.

Education process: OT shares knowledge and expertise about engaging in an occupation with client but client does not actually engage in the occupation during the intervention.

Advocacy: promotes occupational justice and empowers clients to use resources for full participation in occupation

*Supporting health and participation in life through engagement in occupation. The OT's unique contribution is the overarching theme of the domain and the overarching outcome of the process.

Application of the Occupational Therapy Practice Framework to Physical Dysfunction

The occupational therapy process should be conceptualized as a circular process initiated by a referral (Fig. 1-3).

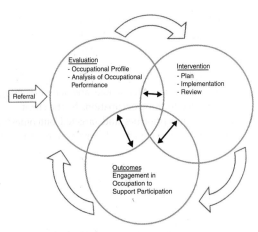

FIGURE 1-3 Intervention process model.

Evaluation

The occupational profile is usually initiated by an interview with the client and significant others in the client's life, and by a thorough review of available records. Interviews may be completed using a formal instrument or informal tools. Although the occupational profile is used to focus subsequent intervention, this profile is often revised throughout the course of intervention to meet a client's needs. The purpose of the occupational profile is to answer the following questions:

1. Who is the client? This requires consideration of not only the individual but includes the significant others in the client's life. In some settings, the client may be identified as a group and not as an individual.
2. Why is the client seeking service? This relates to the occupational needs identified by the individual and significant others.
3. What occupations and activities are successful or problematic for the client? This would also include understanding which occupations are successfully completed by the client.

4. How do contexts and environments influence engagement in occupations and desired outcomes? Some contexts may be supportive whereas others present challenges or prohibit occupational performance.
5. What is the client's occupational history? This includes the level of engagement in various occupations and activities along with the value attributed to those occupations by the client.
6. What are the client's priorities and targeted outcomes? These may be identified as occupational performance, role competence, adaptation to the circumstance, health and wellness, prevention, and/or quality of life issues.

After the occupational profile is developed, the occupational therapist (OT) identifies the necessary additional information to be collected, including areas to be evaluated and which assessment instruments should be used prior to the analysis of occupational performance. The selection of additional information beyond the occupational profile should answer the following questions:

1. What additional data are needed to understand the client's occupational needs, including contextual supports and challenges?
2. What is the best way (most efficient and accurate) to collect these data?
3. How will this information support the intervention plan?
4. How will this information influence potential outcomes?

Intervention Planning

Working with the client, the occupational therapy practitioners (OT and occupational therapy assistant [OTA]) develop a plan using the following approaches or strategies to enhance the client's ability to participate in occupational performance:

- Prevention of disability. This approach is focused on developing the performance skills and patterns that support continued occupational performance and provides interventions that anticipate potential hazards or challenges to occupational performance.

Contextual issues are also addressed using this approach and environmental barriers would be similarly considered.

- Health promotion. A disabling condition is not assumed, but instead occupational therapy services are provided to enhance and enrich occupational pursuits.
- Establish or restore a skill or ability. This strategy is aimed at improving a client's skills or abilities, thus allowing greater participation in occupations.
- Adapt or compensate. This approach is focused on modifying the environment, the activity demands, or the client's performance patterns to support health and participation in occupations.
- Maintain current functional abilities. This approach recognizes that many clients are faced with degenerative disorders, and occupational therapy services should actively address the need to maintain occupational engagement.

The plan includes client-centered goals and methods for reaching them. The values and goals of the client are primary; those of the therapist are secondary. Cultural, social, and environmental factors are incorporated into the plan. The plan must identify the scope and frequency of the intervention and the anticipated date of completion. The outcomes of the intervention must be written at the time the intervention plan is developed. Discharge planning is initiated during the intervention planning process by developing clear outcomes and targeted time frames for completion of goals.

The generation of clear and measurable goals is a very important step in the planning process. Long-term goals or terminal behaviors must reflect a change in occupational performance. For a client to receive authentic occupational therapy services there must be a focus on supporting health and participation in life through engagement in occupation. To meet this outcome, short-term goals or behavioral objectives reflect the incremental steps that must occur to reach this target.

TABLE 1-1   Format for Writing Goals

Goal or Behavior	Step
A. Actor	Begin the goal with a statement such as "Nora will . . .." Name the client as the performer of the action for the goal.
B. Behavior	The occupation, activity, task, or skill to be performed by the client. If this is an outcome or terminal goal, the behavior must reflect occupational performance. Short-term goals or behavioral objectives are often steps to reaching a long-term goal or outcome. A short-term goal or objective may identify a client factor or performance skill as the targeted behavior. An outcome behavior for Nora would be the ability to drive a car, whereas a short-term behavior would be to enter the car and fasten a seatbelt.
C. Condition	The situations for the performance of the stated behavior include social and physical environmental situations for the behavior. Examples of conditions included in a goal are the equipment used, social setting, and training necessary for the stated behavior. In Nora's situation, driving a car with an automatic transmission is far different than driving a car with a manual transmission.
D. Degree	The measure applied to the behavior and the criteria for how well the behavior is performed. These may include repetitions, duration, or the amount of the activity completed. A client may only be expected to complete a small portion of an activity as a short-term goal but the long-term goal would address the targeted occupation. The amount of support provided serves as a measure of degree of behavioral performance. This would include whether the client required minimal assistance, verbal prompts, or performed the task independently. The criteria must be appropriate for the behavior. Safely driving 50% of the time is an inappropriate criterion but using a percentage to indicate that Nora will independently fasten her seat belt 100% of the time provides an appropriate criterion for the behavior
E: Expected time frame	When the goal is to be met, the time period that is anticipated to meet the goal as stated

Adapted from Kettenbach G: Writing SOAP notes, ed 2, Philadelphia, 2004, FA Davis.

Clinical Reasoning Process

Clinical reasoning is defined as the process used by OT practitioners to understand the client's occupational needs, make decisions about intervention services, and think about what we do. There are several forms of clinical reasoning:

- Procedural reasoning is concerned with getting things done, with what has to happen next. The emphasis is often placed on client factors and body functions
- Interactive reasoning is concerned with the interchanges between the client and therapist. The therapist uses this form of reasoning to engage with, understand, and motivate the client.
- Conditional reasoning is concerned with the context in which interventions occur, context in which the client performs

occupations, and how various factors might affect the outcomes and direction of therapy.

- Narrative reasoning uses story making or story telling as a way to understand the client's experience. The client's explanation or description of life and the disability experience reveal themes that permeate the client's understanding that will affect the enactment and outcomes of therapeutic intervention.

Pragmatic reasoning extends beyond the interaction of the client and therapist. This form of reasoning integrates several variables, including the demands of the intervention setting, therapist's competence, client's social and financial resources, and client's potential discharge environment.

BOX 1-2 Questions to Engage in Clinical Reasoning

Procedural Questions
What is the diagnosis?
What prognosis, complications, and other factors are associated with this diagnosis?
What is the general protocol for assessment and intervention with this diagnosis?
What interventions (adjunctive methods, enabling activities, purposeful activities) might be employed?
What evidence supports the use of specific interventions to foster occupational performance?

Interactive Questions
Who is the client?
What are the client's goals, concerns, interests, and values?
How does the client view his or her occupational performance status?
How does the illness or disability fit into the client's performance patterns?
How might I engage this client?
How can we communicate?

Conditional Questions
What contexts has the client identified as important in his or her life?
What future(s) can be imagined for the client?
What events could or would shape the future?
How can I engage the client to imagine, believe in, and work toward a future?

Narrative Reasoning
What does the change in occupational performance mean to this client?
How is this change positioned within the client's life history?
How does the client experience the disabling condition?
What vision does the therapist hold for the client in the future?
What unfolding story will bring this vision to fruition?

Pragmatic Reasoning
What organizational supports and constraints must be incorporated into the provision of services?
What physical environmental factors must be considered when designing an intervention plan?
What is the therapist's knowledge and skill level?

Cultural Competence

The OT should pose the following questions to foster cultural competence in the provision of services:

1. What do I know about the client's culture and beliefs about health?
2. Does the client agree with these beliefs?
3. How will these beliefs influence the intervention and outcomes of services provided?
4. How can the intervention plan support culturally endorsed occupations, roles, and responsibilities to promote the client's engagement in occupation?

Client-Centered Practice

Client-centered practice is guided by the following concepts:

- Language used reflects the client as a person first and the condition second.
- The client is offered choices and supported in directing the occupational therapy process. This requires the occupational therapist to provide information about the client's condition and the evidence available regarding the various types of intervention.
- Intervention is provided in a flexible and accessible manner to meet the client's needs.
- Intervention is contextually appropriate and relevant.
- There is clear respect for differences and diversity in the occupational therapy process.

TABLE 1-2 Comparison of Practice Settings

Practice Setting	Length of Time Services Are Provided	Client Conditions Needing OT Services	Typical OT Approaches Used in Setting	Frequency of Services
			Examples	
Acute care hospitalization	Days to 1 or 2 wk	Acute injuries and illnesses, exacerbations of chronic conditions	Restore ability or skill, modify the activity or context, prevent further disability with an emphasis on discharge setting	Daily
Acute rehabilitation	Weeks	Neurologic, orthopedic, cardiac, general medical conditions	Restore ability or skill, modify the activity or context, prevent further disability with emphasis on occupational performance	Daily (3 hr/day)
Subacute rehabilitation	Weeks to months	Neurologic, orthopedic, cardiac, general medical conditions	Restore ability or skill, modify the activity or context, prevent further disability with emphasis on occupational performance	Daily to weekly
Skilled nursing facilities	Months to years	Neurologic, orthopedic, cardiac, general medical conditions	Restore ability or skill, modify the activity or context, prevent further disability, preserve current skills	Daily, weekly, monthly consultation
Home- and community-based settings	Weeks to months	Neurologic, orthopedic, cardiac, general medical conditions	Restore ability or skill, modify the activity or context, prevent further disability with emphasis on occupational performance	Daily to weekly
Residential care and assisted living units	Months to years	Neurologic, orthopedic, cardiac, general medical conditions	Restore ability or skill, modify the activity or context, prevent further disability, preserve current skills, promote health	Weekly, monthly consultation
Home health care	Weeks to months	Neurologic, orthopedic, cardiac, general medical conditions	Restore ability or skill, modify the activity or context, prevent further disability	Weekly
Outpatient	Weeks to months	Neurologic, orthopedic, cardiac, general medical conditions	Restore ability or skill, modify the activity or context, prevent further disability with emphasis on occupational performance	Weekly
Day treatment	Months to years	Neurologic, orthopedic, cardiac, general medical conditions	Restore ability or skill, modify the activity or context, prevent further disability, preserve current skills, health promotion	Daily, weekly
Work site	Weeks to months	Neurologic, orthopedic, cardiac, general medical conditions	Restore ability or skill, modify the activity or context, prevent further disability with emphasis on occupational performance	Weekly, monthly consultation

Health Promotion and Wellness for People with Physical Disabilities

TABLE 1-3 Selection of Assessments for Use in Health Promotion Physical Disabilities Practice

Assessment Type	Examples
Adjustment scales	Profile of Adaptation to Live Social Support Questionnaire
Other well-being scales	Perceived Well-being Scale
Arthritis	Arthritis McMaster-Toronto Arthritis Patient Reference Disability Questionnaire (MACTAR) Health Assessment Questionnaire (HAQ) Arthritis Impact Measurement Scales (AIMS)
Back pain	Disability Questionnaire
Cancer	Karnofsky Performance Status Measure (KPS) Functional Living Index: Cancer
COPD	American Thoracic Society Respiratory Questionnaire and Grade of Breathlessness Scale
Depression	Beck Depression Inventory
Diabetes	DCCT Questionnaire
Family scales	Caregiver Time-Tradeoff Scale Family Hardiness Inventory
Hardiness scales	Hardiness Scale
Health risks appraisals	The Healthier People Network Risk Appraisal 1999 Youth Risk Behavior Survey
HIV/AIDS	AIDS Health Assessment Questionnaire
Heart	New York Heart Association Functional Classification (NYHA)
Life satisfaction scales	Kansas Family Life Satisfaction Index Index of Life Satisfaction
Multiple sclerosis	Expanded Disability Status Scale
Neurologic head injury	Modified Sickness Impact Profile
Orthopedic	Musculoskeletal Outcomes Data Evaluation and Management System (MO-DEMS)
Pain	MOS Pain Measures
Quality of life	Overall Life Status

Data from Hyner GC, Peterson KW, Travis JW, et al (eds): *Society of prospective medicine handbook of health assessment tools*, Stoughton, WI, 1999, Wellness Associates Publications.

Teaching Activities in Occupational Therapy

Phases of Learning

Learning generally proceeds through three phases. These phases include the acquisition phase, retention phase, and generalization, or transfer, phase. The acquisition, or learning, phase that occurs during initial instruction and practice is often characterized by numerous errors of performance as the learner develops strategies and methods for how to complete the task successfully. The retention phase is demonstrated during subsequent sessions, when the learner demonstrates recall or retention of the task in a similar situation. Transfer of learning, or generalization of skill, is seen when the learner is able to perform the task spontaneously in different environments, such as a client who is able to apply hip precautions correctly at home after learning the precautions in the therapy clinic.

BOX 1-3 Principles of Teaching and Learning in Occupational Therapy

- Identify an activity that has meaning or value to the client and/or family.
- Choose an instructional mode that is compatible with the client's cognition and the characteristics of the task to be taught.
- Organize the learning environment.
- Provide reinforcement and grading of activities.
- Structure feedback and practice schedules.
- Help the client develop self-awareness and self-monitoring skills.

BOX 1-4 Factors That Support Transfer of Learning

- Active participation
- Occupationally embedded instruction
- Intrinsic feedback
- Contextual interference
- Random practice schedules
- Naturalistic contexts
- Whole-task practice
- Strategy development

Documentation of Occupational Therapy Services

TABLE 1-4 Levels of Assistance

Level	Description
Independent	Client is completely independent. No physical or verbal assistance* is required to complete task; task completed safely.
Modified independence	Client is completely independent with task, but may require additional time or adaptive equipment.
Supervised	Client requires supervision to complete task safely; may require a verbal cue for safety.
Contact guard, standby assistance	Hands-on, contact guard assistance is necessary for the client to complete the task safely or caregiver must be within arm's length for safety.
Minimum assistance	Client requires up to 25% physical or verbal assistance of one person to safely complete the task.
Moderate assistance	Client requires 26%-50% physical or verbal assistance of one person to complete the task safely.
Maximal assistance	Client requires 51%-75% physical or verbal assistance of one person to complete the task safely.
Dependent	Client requires more than 75% assistance to complete the task.

*It is important to state whether assistance provided is physical or verbal assistance.

TABLE 1-5 Examples of Short- and Long-Term Goals

Short-Term Goal*	Long-Term Goal†
Client will prepare a cup of tea with minimal verbal assistance for safety and technique.	Client will independently adhere to safety precautions during simple cooking tasks 100% of the time.
Client will brush teeth with moderate physical and verbal assistance while seated at the sink.	Client will complete morning hygiene and grooming independently after task setup while seated at the sink.
Client will don socks with minimal assistance using a sock aide while seated in a wheelchair.	Client will independently complete lower body dressing without assistive devices while seated at the edge of the bed.

*To be completed in 2 weeks.
†To be completed in 4 weeks.

TABLE 1-6 Definitions of Levels of Assistance*

With or Without Helper	FIM Level
No Helper	
7	Complete independence (timely, safety)
6	Modified independence (device)
Helper—Modified Dependence	
5	Supervision (subject = 100%)
4	Minimal assistance (subject ≥ 75%)
3	Moderate assistance (subject ≥ 50%)
Helper—Complete Dependence	
2	Maximal assistance (subject ≥ 25%)
1	Total assistance or not testable (subject < 25%)

*Based on the Functional Independence Measure (FIM). The FIM measures the level of assistance in various domains on a seven-point scale.

BOX 1-5 Fundamental Elements of Documentation

The following elements should be present in all documentation:
1. Client's full name and case number
2. Date and type of occupational therapy contact
3. Identification of type of documentation, agency, and department name
4. Occupational therapy practitioner's signature with a minimum of first name or initial, last name, and professional designation
5. When applicable on notes or reports, signature of recorder directly at the end of the note and the signature
6. Countersignature by an occupational therapist on documentation written by students and occupational therapy assistants when required by law or the facility
7. Acceptable terminology defined within the boundaries of setting
8. Abbreviations usage as acceptable within the boundaries of the setting
9. When no facility requirements are listed, errors corrected by drawing a single line through an error and by initialing the correction (liquid correction fluid and erasures not acceptable)
10. Adherence to professional standards of technology when used to document occupational therapy services
11. Disposal of records within law or agency requirements
12. Compliance with confidentiality standards
13. Compliance with agency or legal requirements of storage of records

From Reitz SM, Austin DJ, Brandt LC: Guidelines to the occupational therapy code of ethics. *Am J Occup Ther* 60:652-658, 2006.

BOX 1-6 Service Provision Terminology

Skilled Terminology
Assess
Analyze
Interpret
Modify
Facilitate
Inhibit
Instruct in:
    compensatory strategies
    hemiplegic dressing techniques
    safety
    adaptive equipment
Fabricate
Design
Adapt
Environmental modifications
Determine
Establish

Unskilled Terminology
Maintain
Help
Watch
Observe
Practice
Monitor

RUMBA

Using a tool such as the RUMBA (also called RHUMBA) test can be beneficial in organizing the therapist's thought process for effective documentation. RUMBA and RHUMBA are acronyms, with each letter identifying something that the therapist should keep in mind when writing goals and documenting the therapeutic process.

- Is the information **R**elevant (the outcome must be relevant)? The goal or outcome must relate to something.
- **H**ow long will it take? Indicate when the goal or outcome will be met.
- Is the information **U**nderstandable? Anyone reading it must know what it means.
- Is the information **M**easurable? There must be a way to know when the goal has been met.
- Is the information **B**ehavioral (describes behaviors)? The goal or outcome must be something that is seen or heard.
- Is the outcome **A**chievable (realistic)? The goal or outcome must be doable and realistic.

The therapist can review the documentation to determine whether these questions are answered, all the while keeping the target audience in mind.

SMART

Another system that may assist the therapist in writing goals is the SMART goals. SMART acronyms stand for significant (and simple), measurable, achievable, related, and time-limited.

- Achieving this goal will make a Significant difference in the client's life.
- You have a clear, Measurable target to aim for and you will know when the client has reached the goal.
- It is reasonable that the client could Achieve this goal in the time allotted.
- Long and short term goals Relate to each other and the goal has a clear connection to the client's occupational needs.
- The goal is Time-limited; short and long term goals have a designated chronological end point.

Infection Control and Safety Issues in the Clinic

BOX 1-7 Summary of Standard Precautions

1. Use extreme care to prevent injuries caused by sharp instruments.
2. Cover minor, nondraining, noninfected skin lesions with an adhesive bandage.
3. Report infected or draining lesions and weeping dermatitis to your supervisor.
4. Avoid personal habits (e.g., nail biting) that increase the potential for oral mucous membrane contact with body surfaces.
5. Perform procedures involving body substances carefully to minimize splatters.
6. Cover environmental surfaces with moisture-proof barriers whenever splattering with body substances might occur.
7. Wash hands regularly, whether or not gloves are worn.
8. Avoid unnecessary use of protective clothing. Use alternate barriers whenever possible.
9. Wear gloves to touch the mucous membrane or nonintact skin of any client, and whenever direct contact with body substances is anticipated.
10. Wear protective clothing (e.g., gown, mask, goggles) when splashing of body substances is anticipated.
11. Ensure that the hospital has procedures for care, cleaning, and disinfection of environmental surfaces and equipment.
12. Handle and process soiled linens so as to minimize the transfer of microorganisms to other patients and environments.
13. Handle used patient-care equipment appropriately to prevent transfer of infectious microorganisms. Ensure that reusable equipment is thoroughly and appropriately cleaned.

BOX 1-8 Technique for Effective Hand Washing

1. Remove all jewelry, except plain band-type rings. Remove watch or move it up. Provide complete access to area to be washed.
2. Approach the sink and avoid touching the sink or nearby objects.
3. Turn on the water and adjust it to a lukewarm temperature and a moderate flow to prevent splashing.
4. Wet your wrists and hands with your fingers directed downward and apply approximately 1 teaspoon of liquid soap or granules.
5. Begin to wash all areas of your hands (palms, sides, backs), fingers, knuckles, and between each finger, using vigorous rubbing and circular motions (Fig. 1-4A). If wearing a band, slide it down the finger a bit and scrub skin underneath it. Interlace fingers and scrub between each finger.
6. Wash for at least 15 seconds, keeping the hands and forearms at elbow level or below, with hands pointed down. Wash longer if you have treated a client known to have an infection.
7. Rinse hands well under running water.
8. Wash wrists and forearms as high as contamination is likely to occur.
9. Rinse hands, wrists, and forearms under running water (see Fig. 1-4B).
10. Use an orangewood stick or nail brush to clean under each fingernail at least once a day when starting work and each time hands are highly contaminated. Rinse nails well under running water (see Fig. 1-4C).
11. Dry your hands, wrists, and forearms thoroughly with paper towels. Use a dry towel for each hand. The water should continue to flow from the tap as you dry your hands.
12. Use another dry paper towel to turn water faucet off (see Fig. 1-4D). Discard all towels in an appropriate container.
13. Use hand lotion as necessary.

Adapted from Zakus SM: *Clinical procedures for medical assistants*, 3rd ed. St. Louis, 1995, Mosby

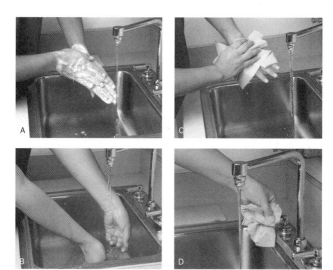

FIGURE 1-4 A, Hand washing technique. Interlace fingers to wash between them. Create a lather with soap. Keep hands pointed down. **B,** Rinse hands well, keeping fingers pointed down. **C,** Use the blunt edge of an orangewood stick to clean under the fingernails. **D,** After drying your hands, turn water faucet off, using a dry paper towel. From Zakus SM: *Clinical procedures for medical assistants*, 3rd ed. St. Louis, 1995, Mosby.

TABLE 1-7 Recommendations for Application of Standard Precautions for Care of All Patients in All Health Care Settings

Component	Recommendations
Hand hygiene	After touching blood, body fluids, secretions, excretions, contaminated items; immediately after removing gloves; between patient contacts
Personal Protective Equipment (PPE)	
Gloves	For touching blood, body fluids, secretions, excretions, contaminated items; for touching mucous membranes and nonintact skin
Gown	During procedures and patient-care activities when contact of clothing or exposed skin with blood or body fluids, secretions, and excretions is anticipated
Mask, eye protection (goggles), face shield*	During procedures and patient-care activities, likely to generate splashes or sprays of blood, body fluids, secretions, especially suctioning, endotracheal intubation
Soiled patient care equipment	Handle in a manner that prevents transfer of microorganisms to others and to the environment; wear gloves if visibly contaminated; perform hand hygiene.
Environmental control	Develop procedures for routine care, cleaning, and disinfection of environmental surfaces, especially frequently touched surfaces in patient care areas.
Textiles and laundry	Handle in a manner that prevents transfer of microorganisms to others and to the environment.
Needles and other sharps	Do not recap, bend, break, or hand-manipulate used needles; if recapping is required, use a one-handed scoop technique only; use safety features when available; place used sharps in puncture-resistant container.
Patient resuscitation	Use mouthpiece, resuscitation bag, other ventilation devices to prevent contact with mouth and oral secretions
Patient placement	Prioritize for single-patient room if patient is at increased risk of transmission, is likely to contaminate the environment, does not maintain appropriate hygiene, or is at increased risk of acquiring infection or developing adverse outcome following infection.
Respiratory hygiene, cough etiquette (source containment of infectious respiratory secretions in symptomatic patients, beginning at initial point of encounter; e.g., triage and reception areas in emergency departments and physician offices)	Instruct symptomatic persons to cover mouth or nose when sneezing or coughing; use tissues and dispose in no-touch receptacle; observe hand hygiene after soiling of hands with respiratory secretions; wear surgical mask if tolerated or maintain spatial separation, >3 ft if possible.

From Siegel JD, Rhinehart E, Jackson M, Chiarello L; Healthcare Infection Control Practices Advisory Committee: *2007 Guideline for isolation precautions: Preventing transmission of infectious agents in healthcare settings*, pp 129-130 (http://www.cdc.gov/hicpac/pdf/isolation/Isolation2007.pdf).

Occupational Performance and the Performance Areas: Evaluation and Intervention

Activities of Daily Living

BOX 2-1 Activities of Daily Living and Instrumental Activities
of Daily Living Categories

Activities of Daily Living (ADLs)
Functional mobility
Self-feeding
Eating (swallowing)
Dressing
Personal hygiene and grooming
Bathing and showering
Bowel and bladder management, toilet hygiene
Sexual activity
Sleep, rest
Personal device care

Instrumental Activities of Daily Living (IADLs)
Care of others, pets, child rearing
Communication management
Community mobility
Financial management
Health management and maintenance
Religious observance
Safety and emergency maintenance
Shopping
Home establishment and management
Meal preparation and cleanup

Levels of Independence

1. Independent: Client can independently perform the activity without cueing, supervision, or assistance, with or without assistive devices, at normal or near-normal speeds. The task is completed safely. If the client requires assistive devices or performs the activity at a slower than customary speed, the term *modified independence* may be used.

2. Supervised: Client requires general supervision (not hands-on) and may require a verbal cue for safety. The occupational therapist (OT) feels comfortable being more than arms' length away at all times.

3. Standby assistance (SBA), contact guard assistance (CGA): Client requires caregiver or someone to provide hands-on guarding to perform a task safely. Note that OTs may tend to use the term *standby assistance* whereas those in other disciplines may use *contact guard assistance*.

4. Minimal assistance: Client requires 25% physical or verbal assistance of one person to complete task safely (client performs 75% or more of the task).

5. Moderate assistance: Client requires 50% physical or verbal assistance of one person to complete task safely (client performs 50% to 74% of the task).

6. Maximal assistance: Client requires physical or verbal assistance for 51% to 75% of activity by one person (client performs 25% to 49% of the task). The helper is doing more than half of the work or task and client is performing less than half.

7. Dependent: Client requires more than 75% physical or verbal assistance (client does less than 25% of the task). For example, he or she can perform only one or two steps of the activity or very few steps of the activity.

Home Safety Checklist

Help prevent falls: Use this list to prioritize work tasks. Leave a copy of this list with the family so they can make further improvements. Note: 32 inch doorway recommendations are for average size person. If overall width of wheelchair or equipment is greater than 28" need 34 to 36" wide door

1. Exterior entrances and exits
- Increase lighting at entry area
- Install stair rails on both sides
- Install door lever handles; double-bolt lock
- Install bevelled, no step, no trip threshold
- Remove screen or storm door if needed
- Create surface to place packages when opening door
- Install peephole on exterior door at level needed for mobility device
- Repair holes, uneven joints on walkway
- Provide non-slip finish to walkway surface/ramps
- Add ramp
  Length _____
  Width _____
  Rails _____
  Platform size _____

2. Interior doors, halls, stairs
- Create clear pathways between rooms
- Apply color contrast or texture change at top and bottom stair edges
- Install door lever handle
- Install swing-clear/off set hinges to widen doorway. Minimum width: 32 inches
- Install bevelled thresholds (max ½ inch)
- Replace or add non-slip surface on steps
- Repair or install stair handrails on both sides
- Clear clutter

3. Bathroom
- Install swing-clear/off set hinges to widen doorway. Minimum width: 32 inches
- Install secure wall reinforcement and place grab bars at toilet, bath and shower
- Install adjustable-height shower head
- Install non-slip strips in bath/shower
- Secure floor bathmat with non-slip, double-sided rug tape
- Elevate toilet height by adding portable seat or raising toilet base on a pedestal
- Adapt flush handle or install flush sensor
- Adapt or relocate toilet paper dispenser
- Round counter corners to provide safety
- Insulate hot water pipes if exposed
- Create sitting knee clearance at basin by removing vanity door and shelves underneath
- Install mirror for sitting or standing view
- Install good-quality non-glare lighting
- Install shower with no threshold if bathing abilities are severely limited
- Install bidet

Recommend : • shower seat • transfer tub bench • 3 in1 commode
  • shower/commode tub slider system • power tub lift • other

4. Kitchen
- Increase task lighting at sink, stove, etc.
- Install D-type cupboard door handles
- Install adjustable shelving to increase access to upper cabinets
- Increase access to under counter storage space by installing pull-out units
- Insulate hot water pipes if exposed
- Install hot-proof surface near oven
- Install switches and outlets at front of counter
- Install pressure-balanced, temperature-regulated, lever faucets
- Create sitting knee clearance under work sites by removing doors or shelves
- Improve color contrast of cabinet and counters surface edges for those with low vision
- Add tactile and color-contrasted controls for those with low vision
- Move microwave to reachable work surface
- Arrange frequently stored items within easy reach given current mobility device and function

FIGURE 2-1 Home safety checklist. (Adapted from Rebuilding Together: Home Safety Checklist; Ralph K. Davies Medical Center: Occupational/Physical Therapy Home Evaluation Form. San Francisco, Ralph K. Davies Medical Center 1993; and Alta Bates Hospital: Occupational Therapy Home Evaluation Form. Albany, Calif, Alta Bates Hospital, 1993.)

Continued

5. Living, dining, bedroom
- Widen or clear pathways within each room by rearranging furniture
- Secure area rug edges with double-sided tape
- Remove throw rugs
- Improve access to and from chairs and beds by inserting risers under furniture legs
- Use side bed rail or chairs with armrests
- Install telephone jack near chair or bed
- Enlarge lamp switch or install touch-control lamp at bedside
- Install adjustable closet rods, shelving and light source for better storage access
- Install vertical pole adjacent to chair and sofa
- Raise furniture to appropriate height using leg extender products
- Install uniform level floor surfaces using wood, tile or low-pile rugs

6. Laundry
- Build a counter for sorting and folding clothes
- Adjust clothesline to convenient height
- Relocate laundry appliances
- Use reacher

7. Telephone and door
- Install phone jacks near bed, sofa, and chair
- Install flashing light or sound amplifier to indicate ringing doorbell for those with visual or hearing problems
- Install mailbox at accessible height

8. Storage space
- Install lights inside closet
- Install adjustable closet rods and shelves
- Install bi-fold or pocket doors

9. Windows
- Install handles and locks that are easy to grip, placed at appropriate heights

10. Electrical outlets and controls
- Install light fixtures or outlet for lamps
- Install switches at top and bottom of stairs

11. Heat, air, light, security, water temp, carbon monoxide controls
- Install smoke/CO detectors, fire extinguishers
- Increase residents' access to environmental control systems
- Ensure water temperature is set at safe temperature (120 degrees Fahrenheit, 49 degrees Celsius) to prevent burns (U.S. Consumer Product Safety Commission, Tap water scalds, Document # 5098 retrieved from http://www.cpsc.gov/cpscpub/pubs/5098.html on August, 26, 2010)

FIGURE 2-1, cont'd

Home Evaluation Checklist

Name _____   Date _____

Address _____

Roles _____

Diagnosis _____

Number of people who live in the home _____

Current mobility status	☐ Independent	☐ needs assist	☐ dependent
Mobility Device used in home:	☐ ambulatory, no device	☐ walker	☐ cane
	☐ power wheelchair	☐ manual wheelchair	

Exterior

Home located on: _____

Type of house	☐ owns home	☐ mobile home	
	☐ apartment	☐ board and care	
Number of floors	☐ one story	☐ split level	☐ two story
Driveway surface	☐ inclined	☐ smooth	
	☐ level	☐ rough	
Is the DRIVEWAY negotiable with current mobility device?	☐ yes	☐ no	
Is the GARAGE accessible?	☐ yes	☐ no	

Entrance

Accessible entrances	☐ front	☐ side	☐ back
Steps	Number_____		
	Height of each_____		
	Width_____		
	Depth_____		
Are there HANDRAILS?	☐ yes	☐ no	
If yes, where are they located?	☐ left	☐ right	

HANDRAIL height from step surface?_____

If no, how much room is available for HANDRAILS? _____

Are landings negotiable?	☐ yes	☐ no

Briefly describe any problems with LANDINGS:

_____

_____

_____

FIGURE 2-1, cont'd

Continued

Ramps	☐ yes	☐ no	
	☐ front	☐ back	
	Height _____		
	Width _____		
	Length_____		
Are there HANDRAILS?	☐ yes	☐ no	
If yes, where are they located?	☐ left	☐ right	Height _____

Condition of current ramp _____

If no ramp, how much room is available for one? _____

Given 1" rise:12" length ratio for ramp, how long should the ramp be? _____

Porch

	Width _____	
	Length_____	
Level at threshold?	☐ yes	☐ no
Lighting available at porch?	☐ yes	☐ no

Door

Width_____

Threshold height _____

Negotiable?	☐ yes	☐ no
	☐ swing in	
	☐ swing out	
	☐ sliding	
Do door locks work?	☐ yes	☐ no
Can door lock be reached with use of current mobility device and can it be safely locked and unlocked considering current status?	☐ yes	☐ no
Type of door knob?	☐ lever	☐ round

Interior

Living Room

| Is furniture arranged for safe maneuverability with current mobility status? | ☐ yes | ☐ no |

Height of frequently used furniture/chair? _____

Type of floor covering: _____

| Able to control TV, phone, lights from seat in living room? | ☐ yes | ☐ no |

Comments _____

FIGURE 2-1, cont'd

Hallways

Can current mobility device be maneuvered in hallway? ☐ yes ☐ no

Hall width _____

Is it adequate for current mobility status? ☐ yes ☐ no

Door width _____

Is it adequate for current mobility status? ☐ yes ☐ no

Sharp turns? ☐ yes ☐ no

Steps? ☐ yes ☐ no   Number _____

Are there HANDRAILS? ☐ yes ☐ no

If yes, where are they located? ☐ left ☐ right   Height _____

Lighting: Is switch within reach with current mobility status? ☐ yes ☐ no

Bedroom

☐ single ☐ shared

Is there room for current mobility device? ☐ yes ☐ no

Type of floor covering? _____

Door:

Width _____

Threshold height _____

Negotiable? ☐ yes ☐ no

☐ swing in ☐ swing out

Bed:

☐ twin ☐ double ☐ queen

☐ king ☐ hospital bed

Overall height _____

Safe and accessible with current mobility status? ☐ yes ☐ no

Would hospital bed fit into room if needed? ☐ yes ☐ no

Able to control TV, phone, lights from bed? ☐ yes ☐ no

Clothing:

Are drawers accessible with current mobility status? ☐ yes ☐ no

Able to reach all items in closet (higher and lower)? ☐ yes ☐ no

Is there adequate lighting in closet? ☐ yes ☐ no

Comments: _____

FIGURE 2-1, cont'd

Continued

Bathroom	☐ private	☐ shared	
Door:			
Width _____			
Swings	☐ in	☐ out	
Will door close with current mobility device inside?	☐ yes	☐ no	
Threshold height _____			
Negotiable?	☐ yes	☐ no	
Tub/Shower	☐ tub/shower combination	☐ shower stall	☐ tub only
Height, floor to rim _____			
Height, inside bottom to rim _____			
Width and length inside	Width _____	Depth _____	
Glass doors?	☐ yes	☐ no	
	☐ sliding	☐ swing	☐ in ☐ out
Width of doors _____			
Handheld shower?	☐ yes	☐ no	
Type of faucet controls	☐ 2 levers	☐ single lever	☐ round
If seated, will user be able to reach faucets?	☐ yes	☐ no	
Is tub/shower accessible safely with current mobility status?	☐ yes	☐ no	
The following equipment is currently being used for bathing in the home	☐ shower seat	☐ transfer tub bench	☐ 3 in1 commode
	☐ shower/commode tub slider system		☐ power tub lift
	☐ shower commode chair		
Is there room for the caregiver to assist?	☐ yes	☐ no	
Sink:			
Height _____		☐ open (no cabinets)	
Faucet type _____		☐ closed (cabinets below)	
Able to reach and use faucet and sink with current mobility status?	☐ yes	☐ no	
Height of mirror _____			
Appropriate height to sit?	☐ yes	☐ no	
Can shelf be reached with current mobility status?	☐ yes	☐ no	
Are hot water pipes insulated?	☐ yes	☐ no	
Type of faucet controls	☐ 2 levers	☐ single lever	☐ round
Electrical outlets within reach from seated or standing position	☐ yes	☐ no	
Comments on clutter/organization? _____			

FIGURE 2-1, cont'd

Toilet:

Height from floor_____

Location of toilet paper_____

Distance from toilet to side wall L _____   R _____

Grab bars: ☐ yes   ☐ no

Location _____

Comments: _____

The following equipment is
currently being used for toileting   ☐ raised toilet seat   ☐ toilet safety rails   ☐ 3 in1 commode

☐ grab bars   ☐ bidet

Kitchen

Door:

Width_____

Threshold height_____

Negotiable?   ☐ yes   ☐ no

Stove:

Height_____

Location of controls   ☐ front   ☐ rear

Able to reach and operate
controls/burners with current
mobility status?   ☐ yes   ☐ no

Oven:

Height from floor to door hinge and door handle _____

Location of oven_____

Is there a nearby surface to rest
hot foods on when removed
from oven?   ☐ yes   ☐ no

Microwave Oven:

Height from floor to door hinge and door handle _____

Location of mircrowave oven _____

Is there a nearby surface to rest
hot foods on when removed
from microwave oven?   ☐ yes   ☐ no

Sink:

Will w/c fit underneath?   ☐ yes   ☐ no

Type of faucet controls   ☐ 2 levers   ☐ single lever   ☐ round

Can faucet be reached while
seated?   ☐ yes   ☐ no

Are hot water pipes insulated?   ☐ yes   ☐ no

FIGURE 2-1, cont'd

Continued

Cupboards:

Height of counters? _____

Accessible from seated position or with current mobility status?	☐ yes	☐ no	
Is there under the counter knee space for a work area?	☐ yes	☐ no	

Refrigerator:

Type:	☐ side by side	☐ freezer on top	☐ freezer on bottom
Hinges on	☐ left	☐ right	
Able to reach all shelves in the refrigerator?	☐ yes	☐ no	
Able to reach all shelves in the freezer?	☐ yes	☐ no	

Switches/outlets:

Able to reach with current mobility status?	☐ yes	☐ no

Lighting:

Adequate in work areas of kitchen?	☐ yes	☐ no

Kitchen table:

Height from floor _____

Will w/c fit under table?	☐ yes	☐ no

Comments: _____

Laundry

Door:

Width _____

Threshold height _____

Negotiable?	☐ yes	☐ no
Steps:	☐ yes	☐ no

Number _____

Height _____

Width _____

Are there HANDRAILS?	☐ yes	☐ no	
If yes, where are they located?	☐ left	☐ right	Height _____
Washer:	☐ Top load	☐ Front load	
Can user reach controls and inside to retrieve clothing?	☐ yes	☐ no	
Dryer:	☐ Top load	☐ Front load	
Can user reach controls and inside to retrieve clothing?	☐ yes	☐ no	

Comments: _____

FIGURE 2-1, cont'd

Safety

Throw rugs	☐ yes	☐ no
Location _____		
Is client and/or family willing to remove?	☐ yes	☐ no
Water Temperature		
Is water temperature set at 120 degrees Fahrenheit?	☐ yes	☐ no
Phone		
Type	☐ programmable ☐ attached to base	☐ cordless	☐ mobile
Within reach of chair?	☐ yes	☐ no
Within reach of bed?	☐ yes	☐ no
Able to retrieve phone, dial and hear caller?	☐ yes	☐ no
Emergency phone numbers posted and programmed into phone?	☐ yes	☐ no
Location _____		
Mailbox		
Able to reach and empty?	☐ yes	☐ no
Location _____		
Doorbell		
Able to identify visitors?	☐ yes	☐ no
Able to hear doorbell?	☐ yes	☐ no
Thermostat		
Able to reach and read controls?	☐ yes	☐ no
Location _____		
Electric outlets/switches		
Height of outlets? _____		
Electrical extension cord hazards?	☐ yes	☐ no
Drapes/Curtains/Blinds		
Able to open with current mobility status?	☐ yes	☐ no
Windows/Doors		
Able to open with current mobility status?	☐ yes	☐ no

FIGURE 2-1, cont'd

Continued

Imperfect floor/floor covering?	☐ yes	☐ no	
Location _____			
Sharp-edged furniture?	☐ yes	☐ no	
Location _____			
Fire extinguisher	☐ yes	☐ no	
Location _____			
Smoke detector	☐ yes	☐ no	
Location _____			
Client hears and understands meaning of smoke detector?	☐ yes	☐ no	
Guns present:	☐ yes	☐ no	
Locked?	☐ yes	☐ no	

Comments on condition of house:

Cleanliness: _____

Disrepair: _____

Clutter issues: _____

Health issues: _____

Equipment present:	☐ shower seat	☐ transfer tub bench	☐ 3 in1 commode
	☐ shower/commode tub slider system		☐ power tub lift
	☐ raised toilet seat	☐ toilet safety rails	☐ grab bars installed
	☐ tub safety rail	☐ shower commode chair	☐ lift recliner chair
	☐ hospital bed with rails	☐ stair glide	

Other equipment/Status of equipment (e.g., borrowed, in disrepair, etc): _____

Problem list: _____

Recommendations for modifications: _____

Equipment recommendations: _____

Patient/Family willing to make modifications:	☐ yes	☐ no
Patient/Family able to make modifications:	☐ yes	☐ no

Cost constraints: _____

Referrals needed: _____

Comments: _____

FIGURE 2-2 Home evaluation checklist. (Adapted from Ralph K. Davies Medical Center: Occupational/Physical Therapy Home Evaluation Form, San Francisco, Ralph K. Davies Medical Center 1993; and Alta Bates Hospital: Occupational Therapy Home Evaluation Form. Albany, Calif, Alta Bates Hospital, 1993.)

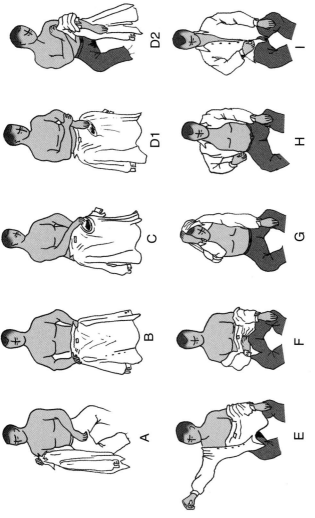

FIGURE 2-3 Steps in donning a shirt, method I. (Courtesy Christine Shaw, Metro Health Center for Rehabilitation, Metro Health Medical Center, Cleveland, Ohio.)

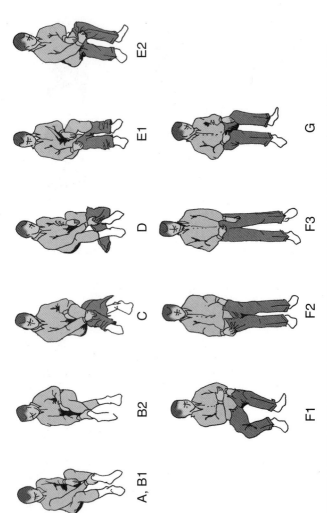

FIGURE 2-4 Steps in donning trousers, method I. (Courtesy Christine Shaw, Metro Health Center for Rehabilitation, Metro Health Medical Center, Cleveland, Ohio.)

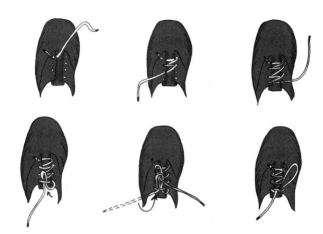

FIGURE 2-5 One-hand shoe-tying method. (Courtesy Christine Shaw, Metro Health Center for Rehabilitation, Metro Health Medical Center, Cleveland, Ohio.)

ONE-HANDED PERSONAL HYGIENE AND GROOMING

1. A hand-held flexible shower hose for bathing and shampooing hair can eliminate the need to stand in the shower and offers the user control of the direction of the spray. The handle can be built up or adapted for limited grasp.

2. A long-handled bath brush or sponge with a soap holder or long cloth scrubber can allow the user to reach legs, feet, and back. A wash mitt and soap on a rope can aid limited grasp. If reach is limited for washing hair, a soft rubber brush with an extended handle or specially designed long-handled adaptive aid can be used to shampoo the hair.

3. A wall-mounted hair dryer may be helpful. This device is useful for clients with limited range of motion (ROM), upper extremity weakness, incoordination, or use of only one upper extremity. The dryer is mounted (wall or stand) to allow the user to manage his or her hair with one arm or position himself or herself to compensate for limited ROM.

4. Long handles on a comb, brush, toothbrush, lipstick, mascara brush, and safety or electric razor may be useful for clients with limited hand to head or hand to face movements. Extensions may be constructed from inexpensive wooden dowels or pieces

of polyvinyl chloride (PVC) pipe found in hardware stores. The handles can be built up or adapted for limited grasp.

5. Spray deodorant, hair spray, and spray powder or perfume can extend the reach by the distance the material sprays.

6. An electric toothbrush and a Water-Pik may be easier to manage than a standard toothbrush; each may need to be adapted for limited grasp.

7. A short reacher can extend reach for using toilet paper. Several types of toilet aids are available in catalogs that sell assistive devices.

8. Dressing sticks can be used to pull garments up after using the toilet. An alternative is the use of a long piece of elastic or webbing with clips on each end that can be hung around the neck and fastened to slacks or panties, preventing them from slipping to the floor during use of the toilet.

9. Safety rails can be used for bathtub transfers, and safety mats or strips can be placed in the bathtub bottom to prevent slipping.

10. A transfer tub bench shower stool or regular chair set in the bathtub or shower stall can eliminate the need to sit on the bathtub bottom or stand to shower, thus increasing safety.

11. Grab bars can be installed to prevent falls and ease transfers.

12. Pump dispensers for shampoo, conditioners, and lotions are easier to manage than containers that require lifting and pouring contents. If using containers that require lifting and pouring, use smaller containers and transfer contents from larger containers to smaller ones.

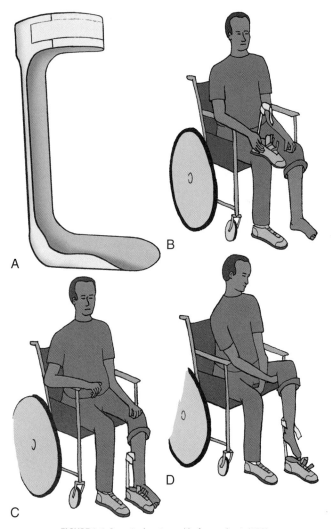

FIGURE 2-6 Steps in donning ankle-foot orthosis (AFO).

Continued

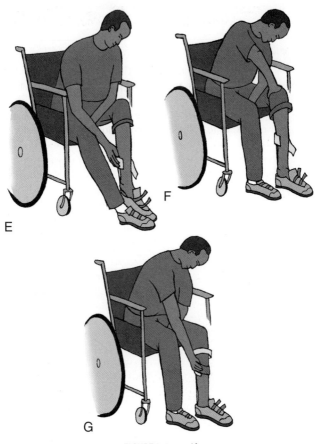

FIGURE 2-6, cont'd

ADLs for Persons with Quadriplegia

DONNING SLACKS (SPINAL CORD INJURY [SCI] LEVEL C6-C7)

1. Long sit on bed with bed rails up. The slacks are positioned at the foot of the bed with the slack legs over the end of the bed, front side up.

2. Sit up and lift one knee at a time by hooking the right hand under right knee to pull the leg into flexion, then put the slacks over the right foot. Return the right leg to extension or semi-extended position while repeating the procedure with the left hand and left knee. If unable to maintain the leg in flexion by holding with one arm or through advantageous use of spasticity, use a dressing band. This device is a piece of elasticized webbing that has been sewn into a figure-of-eight pattern, with one small loop and one large loop. The small loop is hooked around the foot and the large hoop is anchored over the knee. The band is measured for the individual client so that its length is appropriate to maintain the desired amount of knee flexion. Once the slacks are in place, the knee loop is pushed off the knee and the dressing band is removed from the foot with a dressing stick.

3. Work the slacks up the legs, using patting and sliding motions with the palms of the hands.

4. While still sitting, with the slacks to midcalf height, insert the dressing stick in the front belt loop. The dressing stick is gripped by slipping its loop over the wrist. Pull on the dressing stick while extending the trunk, returning to a supine position. Return to a sitting position and repeat this procedure, pulling on the dressing stick and maneuvering the slacks up to thigh level. If balance is adequate, an alternative is for the client to remain sitting and to lean on the left elbow and pull the slacks over the right buttock, and then reverse the process for the other side. Another alternative is for the client to remain in a supine position and roll to one side, throw the opposite arm behind the back, hook the thumb in the waistband, belt loop, or pocket, and pull the slacks up over the hips. These maneuvers can be repeated as often as necessary to get the slacks over the buttocks.

5. Using the palms of the hands in pushing and smoothing motions, straighten the slacks legs.

6. In a supine position, fasten the slacks by hooking the thumb in the loop on the zipper pull, patting the Velcro closed, or using hand splints and buttonhooks if there are buttons or a zipper pull for zippers.

Variation
Substitute the following for step 2. Sit up and lift one knee at a time by hooking the right hand under the right knee to pull the leg into flexion and then cross the foot over the opposite leg above the knee. This position frees the foot to place the slacks more easily and requires less trunk balance. Continue with all the other steps.

REMOVING SLACKS (SCI LEVEL C6-C7)
1. Lying supine in bed with the bed rails up, unfasten the belt and fasteners.
2. Placing the thumbs in the belt loops, waistband, or pockets, work the slacks past the hips by stabilizing the arms in shoulder extension and scooting the body toward the head of the bed.
3. Use the arms as described in step 2 and roll from side to side to get the slacks past the buttocks.
4. Coming to sitting position and alternately pulling the legs into flexion, push the slacks down the legs.
5. The slacks can be pushed off over the feet with a dressing stick or by hooking the thumbs in the waistband.

FRONT OPENING OR PULLOVER GARMENTS (SCI LEVEL C5-C7)
Front opening and pullover garments include blouses, jackets, vests, sweaters, skirts, and front-opening dresses. Upper extremity dressing is frequently performed in the wheelchair for greater trunk stability. The procedure for putting on these garments is as follows.

Donning Front-Opening or Pullover Garments (SCI Level C5-C7)
1. Position the garment across the thighs with the back facing up and the neck toward the knees.
2. Place both arms under the back of the garment and in the armholes.
3. Push sleeves up onto the arms, past the elbows.
4. Using a wrist extension grip, hook the thumbs under the garment back and gather material up from the neck to hem.

5. To pass the garment over the head, adduct and externally rotate the shoulders and flex the elbows while flexing the head forward.

6. When the garment is over the head, relax the shoulders and wrists and remove the hands from the back of the garment. Most of the material will be gathered up at the neck, across the shoulders, and under the arms.

7. To work the garment down over body, shrug the shoulders, lean forward, and use elbow flexion and wrist extension. Use the wheelchair arms for balance, if necessary. Additional maneuvers to accomplish the task are to hook wrists into the sleeves and pull the material free from the underarms, or lean forward, reach back, and slide the hand against the material to aid in pulling the garment down.

8. The garment can be buttoned from the bottom to top with the aid of a buttonhook and wrist-driven flexor hinge splint if hand function is inadequate.

Removing Front Opening or Pullover Garments (SCI Level C5-C7)

1. Sit in the wheelchair and wear wrist-driven flexor hinge splints. Unfasten the buttons (if any) while wearing splints and using a buttonhook. Remove the splints for the remaining steps.

2. For pullover garments, hook the thumb in the back of the neckline, extend the wrist, and pull the garment over the head while turning the head toward the side of the raised arm. Maintain balance by resting against the opposite wheelchair armrest or pushing on the thigh with the extended arm.

3. For stretchy front-opening style clothing, hook the thumb in the opposite armhole and push the sleeve down the arm. Elevation and depression of the shoulders with trunk rotation can be used to get the garment to slip down the arms as far as possible.

4. Hold one cuff with the opposite thumb while the elbow is flexed to pull the arm out of the sleeve.

BRA (BACK-OPENING)

Donning Bra (SCI Level C5-C7)

When worn, this bra style fastens at the back with a hook and eye. The bra is adapted and has loop extenders attached on both the right and left side of the fasteners. Procedurally, the bra is attached in front, first around the body, and then twisted around into position.

The arms are placed in the strap last. Here are the step-by-step directions:

1. Place the bra across the lap with the straps toward the knees and the inside facing up.
2. Using a right to left procedure, hold the end of the bra closest to the right side with the hand or reacher and pass the bra around the back from the right to left side. Lean against bra at the back to hold it in place while hooking the thumb of the left hand in a loop that has been attached near the bra fastener. Hook the right thumb in a similar loop on the right side, and fasten the bra in the front at waist level.
3. Hook the right thumb in the edge of the bra. Using wrist extension, elbow flexion, shoulder adduction, and internal rotation, rotate the bra around the body so that the front of the bra is in front of the body.
4. While leaning on one forearm, hook the opposite thumb in the front end of the strap and pull the strap over shoulder; then repeat the procedure on the other side.

Removing Bra

1. Hook the thumb under the opposite bra strap and push down over the shoulder while elevating the shoulder.
2. Pull the arm out of the strap and repeat the procedure for the other arm.
3. Push the bra down to waist level and turn around as described earlier to bring fasteners to the front.
4. Unfasten the bra by hooking the thumbs into the adapted loops near the fasteners.

Alternatives for a back-opening bra are as follows: (1) a front-opening bra with loops for using a wrist extension grip; or (2) a fully elastic bra that has no fasteners, such as a sports bra, which can be donned like a pullover sweater.

SOCKS

Donning Socks (SCI Level C6-C7)
Method I

1. Sit in wheelchair, or on the bed if balance is adequate, in a cross-legged position, with one ankle crossed over the opposite knee.
2. Pull the sock over the foot using wrist extension and patting movements with the palm of the hand. To prevent pressure

areas, check to make sure that there are no creases or thickened areas on the socks.

Method II

1. Sitting in a wheelchair with the seatbelt fastened, hook one arm at the elbow around the wheelchair upright. This allows for improved stability while reaching.
2. Position the foot on seatbelt stool, chair, or open drawer to elevate the foot easily enough to reach.
3. Pull the sock over the foot using wrist extension and patting movements with the palm of the hand. To prevent pressure areas, check to make sure that there are no creases or thickened areas on the socks.

Method III

1. Use a stocking aid or sock cone to assist in putting on the socks while in this position. Powder the sock cone (to reduce friction) and apply the sock to the cone by using the thumbs and palms of the hands to smooth the sock out on the cone.
2. With the cord loops of sock cone around the wrist or thumb, throw the cone beyond the foot.
3. Maneuver the cone over the toes by pulling the cords, using elbow flexion. Insert the foot as far as possible into the cone.
4. To remove the cone from the sock after the foot has been inserted, move the heel forward off the wheelchair footrest. Use wrist extension (of the hand not operating the sock cone) behind the knee and continue pulling the cords of the cone until it is removed and the sock is in place on the foot. Use the palms to smooth the sock with patting and stroking motions.
5. Two loops can also be sewn onto either side of the top of the sock so that the thumbs can be hooked into the loops and the socks pulled on.

Removing Socks (SCI Level C6-C7)
Method I

1. While sitting in the wheelchair or long sitting in the bed and the hips flexed forward, use a dressing stick or long-handled shoe-horn to push the sock down over the heel. Cross the legs if possible. If an adaptive device is not used, hook the thumb in the socks and use wrist extension to slide the socks off.
2. To protect the skin, use a dressing stick with a coated end to push the sock off the toes.

Method II

1. While long sitting in bed and the hips flexed forward, slide the hands into the socks with the wrist extended, gradually working the sock off the feet and toes.

SHOES

Donning Shoes (SCI Level C6-C7)

1. Use the same position for donning socks as for putting on shoes.
2. Use a long-handled dressing stick and insert it into the tongue of the shoe. Place the shoe opening over the toes. Remove the dressing aid from the shoe and dangle the shoe on the toes.
3. Using the palm of the hand on the sole of the shoe, pull the shoe toward the heel of the foot. One hand is used to stabilize the leg while the other hand pushes against the sole of the shoe to work the shoe onto the foot. Use the palms and sides of the hand to push the shoe on.
4. With the feet flat on the floor or on the wheelchair footrest and the knees flexed 90 degrees, place a long-handled shoehorn in the heel of the shoe and press down on top of the flexed knee until the heel is in the shoe.
5. Fasten the shoes.

Removing Shoes (SCI Level C6-C7)

1. Sitting in the wheelchair with the legs crossed, as described earlier, unfasten the shoes.
2. Use the shoehorn or dressing stick to push on the heel counter of the shoe, dislodging it from the heel. The shoe will drop or can be pushed to the floor with the dressing stick.

Feeding Activities

Feeding may be assisted by a variety of devices, depending on the level of muscle function. Someone with an injury from C1-C4 will likely need assistance to eat unless an electric self-feeding device is used. Once set up, these devices allow independence by using head movement to hit a switch that turns the plate and brings the spoon down to the plate and back up to mouth level.

An injury at C5 may require mobile arm supports or externally powered splints and braces. A wrist splint and universal cuff may be used together if a wrist-driven flexor hinge splint is not used.

The universal cuff holds the eating utensil and the splint stabilizes the wrist. A nonskid mat and a plate with a plate guard may provide adequate stability of the plate for pushing and picking up food (C5-C7).

A regular or swivel spoon-fork combination with a universal cuff can be used when there is minimal muscle function (C5). A long plastic straw with a straw clip to stabilize it in the cup or glass eliminates the need for picking up the cups. A bilateral or unilateral clip-type holder on a glass or cup makes it possible for many persons with hand and arm weakness to manage liquids without a straw.

Built-up utensils may be useful for those with some functional grasp or tenodesis grasp. Food may be cut with an adapted knife if arm strength is adequate to manage the device. Food may also be cut using a sharp knife if a wrist-driven flexor hinge splint is used.

Personal Hygiene and Grooming

1. Use a padded shower seat or padded transfer tub bench and transfer board for transfers (SCI level C1-C7).
2. Extend reach by using long-handled bath sponges with a loop handle or built-up handle (SCI level C6-C7).
3. Eliminate the need to grasp the washcloth by using bath mitts or bath gloves (SCI level C5-C7).
4. Hold comb and toothbrush with a universal cuff (SCI level C5-C7).
5. Use a wall-mounted hair dryer. Use a universal cuff to hold the brush or comb for hair styling while using the mounted hair dryer (SCI level C5-C7).
6. Use a clip-type holder for an electric razor (SCI level C5-C7).
7. Persons with quadriplegia can use suppository inserters to manage bowel care independently (SCI level C6-C7).
8. Use a skin inspection mirror with a long stem and looped handle for independent skin inspection. Devices and methods selected must be adapted according to the degree of weakness of each client (SCI level C6-C7).
9. Adapted leg bag clamps to empty catheter leg bags are also available for individuals with limited hand function. Elastic leg bag straps may also be replaced with Velcro straps (SCI level C5-C7).

10. If the client is unable to reach the leg back clamp, a commercially available electric leg bag clamp allows the individual to drive up to a urinal and empty the leg back with the switch of a button (Richardson products; SCI level C1-C7).

Mobility

BOX 2-2   Questions to Ask Before Making Specific Recommendations for a Wheelchair

- Who will pay for the wheelchair?
- Who will determine the preferred durable medical equipment (DME) provider, the insurance company, client, or therapist?
- What is the specific disability?
- What is the prognosis?
- Is range of motion limited?
- Is strength or endurance limited?
- How will the client propel the chair?
- How old is the client?
- How long is the client expected to use the wheelchair?
- What was the client's lifestyle and how has it changed?
- Is the client active or sedentary?
- How will the dimensions of the chair affect the client's ability to transfer to various surfaces?
- What is the maneuverability of the wheelchair in the client's home or community (e.g., entrances and egress, door width, turning radius in bathroom and hallways, floor surfaces)?
- What is the ratio of indoor to outdoor activities?
- Where will the wheelchair be primarily used—in the home, at school, at work, or in the community?
- Which mode of transportation will be used? Will the client be driving a van from the wheelchair? How will it be loaded and unloaded from the car?
- Which special needs (e.g., work heights, available assistance, accessibility of toilet facilities, parking facilities) are recognized in the work or school environment?
- Does the client participate in indoor or outdoor sports activities?
- How will the wheelchair affect the client psychologically?
- Can accessories and custom modifications be medically justified, or are they luxury items?
- What resources does the client have for equipment maintenance (e.g., self, family, caregivers)?

Wheelchair Selection

MANUAL VERSUS ELECTRIC OR POWER WHEELCHAIRS

Manual Wheelchair

- Does the user have sufficient strength and endurance to propel the chair at home and in the community over varied terrain?
- Does manual mobility enhance functional independence and cardiovascular conditioning of the wheelchair user?
- Will the caregiver be propelling the chair at any time?
- What will be the long-term effects of the propulsion choice?

Power Chairs

- Does the user demonstrate insufficient endurance and functional ability to propel a manual wheelchair independently?
- Does the user demonstrate progressive functional loss, making powered mobility an energy-conserving option?
- Is powered mobility needed to increase independence at school, at work, and in the community?
- Does the user demonstrate cognitive and perceptual ability to operate a power-driven system safely?
- Does the user or caregiver demonstrate responsibility for care and maintenance of the equipment?
- Is a van available for transportation?
- Is the user's home accessible for use of a power wheelchair?
- Has the user been educated regarding the rear, mid, and front wheel drive systems and been guided objectively in making the appropriate selection?

MANUAL RECLINE VERSUS POWER RECLINE VERSUS TILT WHEELCHAIRS

Manual Recline Wheelchair

- Is the client unable to sit upright because of hip contractures, poor balance, or fatigue?
- Is a caregiver available to assist with weight shifts and position changes?
- Is relative ease of maintenance a concern?
- Is cost a consideration?

Power Recline Versus Tilt Wheelchair

- Does the client have the potential to operate independently?
  - Are independent weight shifts and position changes indicated for skin care and increased sitting tolerance?
  - Does the user demonstrate safe and independent use of controls?
  - Are there resources for care and maintenance of the equipment?
  - Does the user have significant spasticity that is facilitated by hip and knee extension during the recline phase?
  - Does the user have hip or knee contractures that prohibit her or his ability to recline fully?
  - Will a power recline or tilt decrease or make more efficient use of caregiver time?

- Will a power recline or tilt feature on the wheelchair reduce the need for transfers to the bed for catheterizations and rest periods throughout the day?
- Will the client require quick position changes in the event of hypotension and/or dysreflexia?
- Has a reimbursement source been identified for this add-on feature?

FOLDING VERSUS RIGID MANUAL WHEELCHAIRS

Folding Wheelchairs

- Is the folding frame needed for transport, storage, or home accessibility?
- Which footrest style is necessary for transfers, desk clearance, and other daily living skills? Elevating footrests are available only on folding frames.
- Is the client or caregiver able to lift, load, and fit the chair into necessary vehicles?
- Equipment suppliers should have knowledge and a variety of brands available. Frame weight can range from approximately 28 to 50 lb, depending on size and accessories. Frame adjustments and custom options depend on the model.

Rigid Wheelchairs

- Does the user or caregiver have the upper extremity function and balance to load and unload the nonfolding frame from a vehicle if driving independently?
- Will the user benefit from the improved energy efficiency and performance of a rigid frame?

LIGHTWEIGHT (FOLDING OR NONFOLDING) VERSUS STANDARD-WEIGHT (FOLDING) WHEELCHAIRS

Lightweight Wheelchairs: Under 35 Pounds

- Does the user have the trunk balance and equilibrium necessary to handle a lighter frame weight?
- Does the lighter weight enhance mobility by reducing the user's fatigue?
- Will the user's ability to propel the chair or handle parts be enhanced by a lighter weight frame?
- Are custom features (e.g., adjustable height back, seat angle, axle mount) necessary?

Standard-Weight Wheelchairs: More Than 35 Pounds

- Does the user need the stability of a standard-weight chair?
- Does the user have the ability to propel a standard-weight chair?
- Can the caregiver manage the increased weight when loading the wheelchair and fitting into a vehicle?
- Will the increased weight of parts be unimportant during daily living skills?
- Custom options are limited, and these wheelchairs are usually less expensive (except heavy-duty models required for users more than 250 lb).

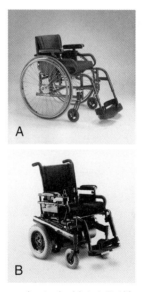

FIGURE 2-7 Manual versus electric wheelchair. **A,** Rigid frame chair with swing-away footrests. **B,** Power-driven wheelchair with hand control. (**A,** Courtesy Quickie Designs, Fresno, Calif; **B,** courtesy Invacare Corporation, Elyria, Ohio.)

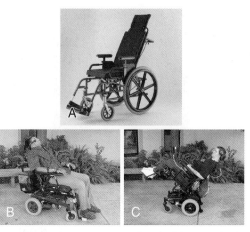

FIGURE 2-8 Manual recline versus power recline wheelchair. **A,** Reclining back on folding frame. **B,** Low-shear power recline with collar mount chin control on electric wheelchair. **C,** Tilt system with head control on electric wheelchair. (**A,** Courtesy Quickie Designs, Fresno, Calif; **B** and **C,** courtesy Luis Gonzalez.)

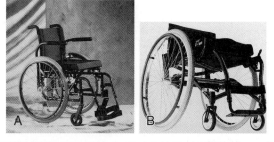

FIGURE 2-9 Folding versus rigid wheelchair. **A,** Lightweight folding frame with swing-away footrests. **B,** Rigid aluminum frame with tapered front end and solid foot cradle. (**A,** Courtesy Quickie Designs, Fresno, Calif; **B,** courtesy Invacare Corporation, Elyria, Ohio.)

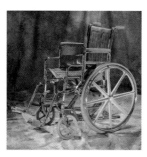

FIGURE 2-10 Standard folding frame (more than 35 lb) with swing-away footrests. (Courtesy Everest & Jennings, Inc.)

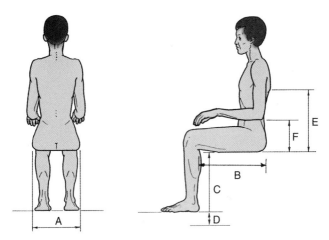

FIGURE 2-11 Measurements for wheelchairs. **A,** Seat width. **B,** Seat depth. **C,** Seat height from floor. **D,** Footrest clearance. **E,** Back height. **F,** Armrest height. (Adapted from Wilson A, McFarland SR: *Wheelchairs: A prescription guide.* Charlottesville, Va, Rehabilitation Press, 1986.)

Transfer Techniques

GUIDELINES FOR USING PROPER MECHANICS

The therapist should be aware of the following principles of basic body mechanics:

1. Get close to the client or move the client close to you.
2. Position your body to face the client (face head on).
3. Bend the knees; use your legs, not your back.
4. Keep a neutral spine (not bent or arched back).
5. Keep a wide base of support.
6. Keep your heels down.
7. Don't tackle more than you can handle; ask for help.
8. Don't combine movements. Avoid rotating at the same time as bending forward or backward.

The therapist should consider the following questions before performing a transfer:

1. What medical precautions affect the client's mobility or method of transfer?
2. Can the transfer be performed safely by one person, or is assistance required?
3. Has enough time been allotted for safe execution of a transfer? Are you in a hurry?
4. Does the client understand what is going to happen? If not, does he or she demonstrate fear or confusion? Are you prepared for this limitation?
5. Is the equipment (e.g., wheelchair, bed) that the client is being transferred to and from in good working order and in a locked position?
6. What is the height of the bed (or surface) in relation to the wheelchair? Can the heights be adjusted so that they are similar? Transferring downhill is easier than uphill.
7. Is all equipment placed in the correct position?
8. Is all unnecessary bedding and equipment (e.g., footrests, armrests) moved out of the way so that you are working without obstructions?
9. Is the client dressed properly in case you need to use a waistband to assist? If not, do you need a transfer belt or other assistance?

10. What are the other components of the transfer, such as leg management and bed mobility?

PRINCIPLES OF BODY POSITIONING

Pelvic Tilt

Generally, after the acute onset of a disability or prolonged time spent in bed, clients assume a posterior pelvic tilt (i.e., a slouched position with lumbar flexion). In turn, this posture moves the center of mass back toward the buttocks. The therapist may need to cue verbally or assist the client manually into a neutral or slightly anterior pelvic tilt position to move the center of mass forward over the center of the client's body and over the feet in preparation for the transfer.

Trunk Alignment

It may be observed that the client's trunk alignment is shifted to the right or left side. If the therapist assists in moving the client while the client's weight is shifted to one side, the movement could throw the client and therapist off balance. The client may need verbal cues or physical assistance to come to and maintain a midline trunk position before and during the transfer.

Weight Shifting

The transfer is initiated by shifting the client's weight forward, removing weight from the buttocks. This movement allows the client to stand, partially stand, or be pivoted by the therapist. This step must be performed regardless of the type of transfer.

Lower Extremity Positioning

The client's feet must be placed firmly on the floor with the ankles stabilized and the knees aligned at 90 degrees of flexion over the feet. This position allows the weight to be shifted easily onto and over the feet. Heels should be pointing toward the surface to which the client is transferring. The client should be barefoot or have shoes on to prevent slipping out of position. Shoes with proper ankle support are beneficial with patients who have weakness or instability in their ankles or feet. The feet can easily pivot in this position, and the risk of twisting or injuring an ankle or knee is minimized.

Upper Extremity Positioning

The client's arms must be in a safe position or in a position in which he or she can assist in the transfer. If one or both of the upper extremities is nonfunctional, the arms should be placed in a safe position that will not be in the way during the transfer (e.g., in the client's lap). If the client has partial or full movement, motor control, or strength, she or he can assist in the transfer by reaching toward the surface to be reached or by pushing off from the surface to be left. The decision to request the client to use the arms during the transfer is based on the therapist's prior knowledge of the client's motor function. The client should be encouraged not to reach or grab for the therapist during the transfer because this could throw balance off.

PREPARING EQUIPMENT AND CLIENT FOR TRANSFER

The transfer process includes setting up the environment, positioning the wheelchair, and helping the client into a pretransfer position. The following is a general overview of these steps.

Positioning the Wheelchair

1. Place the wheelchair at approximately a 0- to 30-degree angle to the surface to which the client is transferring. Note that the angle depends on the type of transfer and the client's level of assist.
2. Lock the brakes on the wheelchair and the bed.
3. Place both of the client's feet firmly on the floor, hip width apart, with the knees over the feet.
4. Remove the wheelchair armrest closer to the bed.
5. Remove the wheelchair pelvic seatbelt.
6. Remove the wheelchair chest belt and trunk or lateral supports, if present.

Bed Mobility in Preparation for Transfer
Rolling the Client Who has Hemiplegia

1. Before rolling the client, you may need to put your hand under the client's scapula on the weaker side and gently mobilize it forward (into protraction) to prevent the client from rolling onto the shoulder, potentially causing pain and injury.
2. Assist the client in clasping the strong hand around the wrist of the weak arm, and lift the upper extremities upward toward the ceiling.

3. Assist the client in flexing his or her knees.
4. You may assist the client to roll onto her or his side by first moving the arms toward the side, then the legs, and finally by placing one of the therapist's hand at the scapula area and the other therapist's hand at the hip, guiding the roll.

Side-Lying to Sit Up at the Edge of Bed
1. Bring the client's feet off the edge of the bed.
2. Stabilize the client's lower extremities with your knees.
3. Shift the client's body to an upright sitting position.
4. Place the client's hands on the bed at the sides of his or her body to help maintain balance.

Scooting to the Edge of the Bed
When working with a client who has sustained a stroke or traumatic brain injury, walk the client's hips toward the edge of the bed. Shift the client's weight to the less or unaffected side, position your hand behind the opposite buttock, and guide the client forward. Then shift the client's weight to the more affected side, and repeat the procedure if necessary. Move forward until the client's feet are flat on the floor.

In the case of an individual with a spinal cord injury, grasp her or his legs from behind the knees and gently pull the client forward, placing the client's feet firmly on the floor and making sure that the ankles are in a neutral position.

Types of Transfers
Stand Pivot Transfers
The standing pivot transfer requires the client to be able to come to a standing position and pivot on both feet. It is most commonly used with clients who have hemiplegia, hemiparesis, or a general loss of strength or balance. If the client has significant hemiparesis, stand pivot transfers encourage the less or unaffected side to accommodate most of the body weight and may put the more affected limb (ankle) at risk while pivoting.

Wheelchair to Bed or Mat Transfer
1. Facilitate the client to scoot to the edge of the surface and put his or her feet flat on the floor. The client's heels should be pointed toward the surface to which the client is transferring. The feet should not be perpendicular to the transfer surface but the heel should be angled toward the surface.

2. Stand on the client's affected side with your hands on the client's scapulae or around the client's trunk, waist, or hips. Stabilize the client's involved foot and knee with your own foot and knee. Provide assistance by guiding the client forward as the buttocks are lifted up from the present surface and toward the transfer surface.
3. The client reaches toward the surface to which he or she is transferring or pushes off the surface from which he or she is transferring.
4. Guide the client toward the transfer surface and gently help her or him down to a sitting position.

Variations: Stand Pivot and/or Stand-Step Transfer

A stand pivot and/or stand-step transfer is generally used when a client can take small steps toward the surface goal and not just pivot toward the transfer surface. The therapist's intervention may range from physical assistance to accommodate for potential loss of balance to facilitation of near-normal movement, equal weight bearing, and maintenance of appropriate posture for clients with hemiplegia or hemiparesis. If a client demonstrates impaired cognition or a behavior deficit, including impulsiveness and poor safety judgment, the therapist may need to provide verbal cues or physical guidance.

Sliding Board Transfers

Sliding board transfers are best used with those who cannot bear weight on the lower extremities and who have paralysis, weakness, or poor endurance in their upper extremities. If the client is going to assist the caregiver in this transfer, the client should have good upper extremity strength. It is most often used with persons who have lower extremity amputations, those with SCIs, or bariatric clients.

Method

1. Position and set up the wheelchair as outlined earlier.
2. Lift the leg closer to the transfer surface and place the board under this leg, midthigh between the buttocks and knee, angled toward the opposite hip. The board must be firmly under the thigh and firmly on the surface to which the client is transferring.
3. Block the client's knees with your own knees.
4. Instruct the client to place one hand toward the edge of the board and the other hand on the wheelchair seat.

5. Instruct the client to lean forward and slightly away from the transferring surface.
6. The client should transfer his or her upper body weight in the direction opposite to which he or she is going. The client should use both arms to lift or slide the buttocks along the board.
7. Assist the client where needed to shift weight and support the trunk while moving to the intended surface.

Bent Pivot Transfer: Bed to Wheelchair

The bent pivot transfer is used when the client cannot initiate or maintain a standing position. A therapist often prefers to keep a client in the bent knee position to maintain equal weight bearing, provide optimal trunk and lower extremity support, and perform a safer and easier therapist-assisted transfer.

Method

1. Assist the client to scoot to the edge of the bed until both of the client's feet are flat on the floor. Grasp the client around the waist, trunk, hips, or even under the buttocks if a moderate or maximal amount of assistance is required.
2. Facilitate the client's trunk into a midline position.
3. Shift the weight forward from the buttocks toward and over the client's feet.
4. Have the client reach toward the surface to which she or he is transferring or push from the surface from which he or she is transferring.
5. Assist the client by guiding and pivoting the client around toward the transfer surface

   Depending on the amount of assistance required, the pivoting portion can be done in two or three steps, with the therapist repositioning himself or herself and the client's lower extremities between steps. The therapist has a variety of choices of where to hold or grasp the client during the bent pivot transfer, depending on the weight and height of the client in relation to the therapist and client's ability to assist in the transfer. Variations include using both hands and arms at the waist, or trunk, or one or both hands under the buttocks. The therapist never grasps under the client's weak arm or grasps the weak arm, an action that could cause significant injury because of weak musculature and poor stability around the shoulder girdle. The choice is made with consideration to proper body mechanics. Trial and error of technique is advised to allow for optimal facilitation of client independence, safety, and the therapist's proper body mechanics.

Dependent Transfers

The dependent transfer is designed for use with the client who has minimal to no functional ability. If this transfer is performed incorrectly, it is potentially hazardous for the therapist and client. This transfer should be practiced with able-bodied persons and initially used with the client only when another person is available to assist.

The purpose of the dependent transfer is to move the client from surface to surface. The requirements are that the client be cooperative and willing to follow instructions. The therapist should be keenly aware of correct body mechanics and his or her own physical limitations. With heavy clients, it is always best to use the two-person transfer, or at least to have a second person available to spot the transfer.

One-Person Dependent Sliding Board Transfer

The procedure for transferring the client from wheelchair to bed is as follows:

1. Set up the wheelchair and bed as described earlier.
2. Position the client's feet together on the floor, directly under the knees, and swing the outside footrest away. Grasp the client's legs from behind the knees and pull the client slightly forward in the wheelchair so that the buttocks will clear the large wheel when the transfer is made.
3. Place a sliding board under the client's inside thigh, midway between the buttocks and the knee, to form a bridge from the bed to the wheelchair. The sliding board is angled toward the client's opposite hip.
4. Stabilize the client's feet by placing your feet laterally around the client's feet.
5. Stabilize the client's knees by placing your own knees firmly against the anterolateral aspect of the client's knees.
6. Facilitate the client to lean over the knees by guiding him or her forward from the shoulders. The client's head and trunk should lean opposite the direction of the transfer. The client's hands can rest on his or her lap.
7. Reach under the client's outside arm and grasp the waistband of the trousers or under the buttocks. On the other side, reach over the client's back and grasp the waistband or under the buttocks.

8. After your arms are positioned correctly, lock them to stabilize the client's trunk. Keep your knees slightly bent and brace them firmly against the client's knees.

9. Gently rock with the client to gain some momentum, and prepare to move after the count of three. Count to three aloud with the client. On three, holding your knees tightly against the client's knees, transfer the client's weight over his or her feet. You must keep your back straight and your knees bent to maintain good body mechanics.

10. Pivot with the client and move him or her onto the sliding board. Reposition yourself and the client's feet and repeat the pivot until the client is firmly seated on the bed surface, perpendicular to the edge of the mattress and as far back as possible. This step usually can be achieved in two or three stages.

11. You can secure the client on the bed by easing him or her against the back of an elevated bed or on the mattress in a side-lying position, and then by lifting the legs onto the bed.

The one-person dependent sliding board transfer can be adapted to move the client to other surfaces. It should be attempted only when therapist and client feel secure with the wheelchair to bed transfer.

Two-Person Dependent Transfers

Bent Pivot: With or Without a Sliding Board Bed to Wheelchair. A bent pivot transfer is used to allow increased therapist interaction and support. It allows the therapist greater control of the client's trunk and buttocks during the transfer. This technique can also be used during a two-person dependent transfer. It is often used with neurologically involved clients because trunk flexion and equal weight bearing are often desirable with this diagnosis. The steps in this two-person procedure are as follows:

1. Set up the wheelchair and bed as described earlier.
2. One therapist assumes a position in front of the client and the other in back.
3. The therapist in front assists in walking the client's hips forward until the feet are flat on the floor.
4. The same therapist stabilizes the client's knees and feet by placing his or her knees and feet lateral to each of the client's.

5. The therapist in back positions himself or herself squarely behind the client's buttocks, grasping the client's waistband or the sides of the client's slacks, or placing his or her hands under the buttocks. Maintain proper body mechanics.

6. The therapist in front moves the client's trunk into a midline position, grasps the client around the back of the shoulders, waist, or hips, and guides the client to lean forward and shift his or her weight forward, over the feet and off the buttocks. The client's head and trunk should lean in the direction opposite the transfer. The client's hands can rest on the lap.

7. As the therapist in front shifts the client's weight forward, the therapist in back shifts the client's buttocks in the direction of the transfer. This can be done in two or three steps, making sure that the client's buttocks land on a safe, solid surface. The therapists reposition themselves and the client to maintain safe and proper body mechanics.

8. The therapists should be sure they coordinate the time of the transfer with the client and one another by counting to three aloud and instructing the team to initiate the transfer on three.

9. Transfer or gait belts may be used to offer a place to grasp while assisting the client in a transfer. The belt is placed securely around the waist and often used instead of the client's waistband. The belt should not be allowed to slide up the client's trunk as leverage will be compromised.

Work Evaluation and Work Programs

BOX 2-3 Twenty Physical Demands of Work

Balancing
Carrying
Climbing
Crawling
Crouching
Feeling
Fingering
Handling
Hearing
Kneeling
Lifting
Pulling
Pushing
Reaching
Seeing
Sitting
Standing
Stooping
Talking
Walking

Data from U.S. Department of Labor, Employment and Training Administration: *Revised dictionary of occupational titles*, vols. I and II, 4th ed. Washington, DC, U.S. Government Printing Office, 1991.

TABLE 2-1 Definitions for Overall Level of Work

Level of Work	Definition
Sedentary	Exerting up to 10 lb of force occasionally, a negligible amount of force frequently to lift, carry, push, pull, or otherwise move objects, including the human body. Sedentary work involves sitting most of the time, but may involve walking or standing for brief periods of time. Jobs are sedentary if walking and standing are required only occasionally, but all other sedentary criteria are met.
Light	Exerting up to 20 lb of force occasionally, up to 10 lb of force frequently, or a negligible amount of force constantly to move objects. Physical demand requirements are in excess of those for sedentary work. Even though the weight lifted may be only a negligible amount, a job should be rated light work: (1) when it requires walking or standing to a significant degree; (2) when it requires sitting most of the time, but entails pushing or pulling of arm or leg controls; or (3) when the job requires working at a production rate pace entailing the constant pushing or pulling of materials even though the weight of those materials is negligible. **NOTE:** The constant stress and strain of maintaining a production rate pace, especially in an industrial setting, can be and is physically demanding of a worker, even though the amount of force exerted is negligible.
Medium	Exerting 20-50 lb of force occasionally, 10-25 lb of force frequently, or greater than negligible up to 10 lb of force constantly to move objects. Physical demand requirements are in excess of those for light work.
Heavy	Exerting 50-100 lb of force occasionally, 25-50 lb of force frequently, or 10-20 lb of force constantly to move objects. Physical demand requirements are in excess of those for medium work.
Very heavy	Exerting force in excess of 100 lb of force occasionally, in excess of 50 lb of force frequently, or in excess of 20 lb of force constantly to move objects. Physical demand requirements are in excess of those for heavy work.

TABLE 2-2 Definitions for Physical Demand Frequencies

Physical Demand Frequency	Definition
Never	Activity or condition does not exist
Occasionally	Up to ⅓ of the day
Frequently	⅓ to ⅔ of the day
Constantly	⅔ to full day

Data from U.S. Department of Labor, Employment and Training Administration: *Revised dictionary of occupational titles*, vols. I and II, 4th ed. Washington, DC, U.S. Government Printing Office, 1991; U.S. Department of Labor, Employment and Training Administration: *The revised handbook for analyzing jobs.* Indianapolis, Ind, JIST Works, 1991

TABLE 2-3 Strength Demands of Work

	Frequency of Force Exertion or Weight Carried		
Strength Rating	Occasional Up to ⅓ of the day	Frequent ⅓ to ⅔ of the day	Constant Over ⅔ of the day
Sedentary	10 lb	Negligible	Negligible
Light	20 lb	10 lb	Negligible
Medium	20-50 lb	10-25 lb	10 lb
Heavy	50-100 lb	25-50 lb	10-20 lb
Very heavy	Over 100 lb	50-100 lb	20-50 lb

Data from U.S. Department of Labor, Employment and Training Administration: *Revised dictionary of occupational titles*, vols. I and II, 4th ed. Washington, DC, U.S. Government Printing Office, 1991.

TABLE 2-4 High-Risk Repetition Rates for the Upper Extremity

Body Part	Repetitions Per Minute
Shoulder	More than 2.5
Upper arm, elbow	More than 10
Forearm, wrist	More than 10
Finger	More than 200

From Kilborn A: Repetitive work of the upper extremity. Part II: The scientific basis for the guide. *Int J Ind Ergonomics* 14:59-86, 1994.

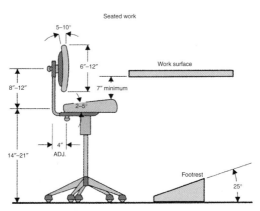

Optimal work surface height varies with performed:
Precision work = 31–37 inches
Reading/writing = 28–31 inches
Typing/light assembly = 21–28 inches
Seat and back rest heights should be adjustable as noted in chair requirements

A

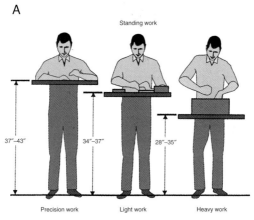

Workbench heights should be:
Above elbow height for precision work
Just below elbow height for light work
4–6 inches below elbow height for heavy work

B

FIGURE 2-12 Recommended dimensions of workstations. **A,** Seated work. **B,** Standing work. (From Cohen AL, Gjessing CC, Fine LJ, et al: *Elements of ergonomics programs: A primer based on workplace evaluations of musculoskeletal disorders* (DHHS [NIOSH] Publ. No. 97-117). Washington DC, U.S. Government Printing Office, 1997.)

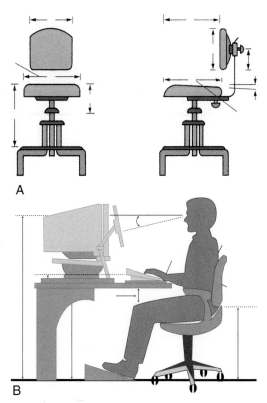

FIGURE 2-13 A, Recommended chair characteristics. Dimensions are given using both front and side views for width (A), depth (E), vertical adjustability (D), and angle (I) and for backrest width (C), height (F), and vertical (H) and horizontal (G) adjustability relative to the chair seat. The angle of the backrest should be adjustable horizontally from 12-17 inches (30-43 cm), by either a slide-adjust or a spring, and vertically from 7-10 inches (18-25 cm). The adjustability is needed to provide back support during different types of seated work. The seat should be adjustable within at least a 6-inch (15-cm) range. The height above the floor of the chair seat with this adjustment range will be determined by the workplace, with or without a footrest. **B,** Proper seated position for computer user. (**A** from Eggleton E (ed): *Ergonomic design for people at work,* vol 1. New York, Van Nostrand Reinhold, 1983; **B** from U.S. Department of Labor, Occupational Safety and Health Administration: *Working safely with video display terminals,* 1997 (www.osha.gov/ Publications/osha3092.pdf).)

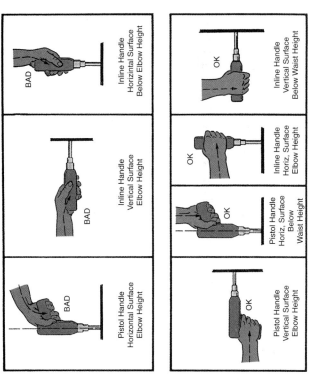

FIGURE 2-14 Hand tool design and wrist posture. (From Armstrong T: *An ergonomic guide to carpal tunnel syndrome.* Akron, Ohio, American Industrial Hygiene Association, 1983.)

General Ergonomic Risk Analysis Checklist

Check the box if your answer is "yes" to the question. A "yes" response indicates that an ergonomic risk factor that requires further analysis may be present.

Manual Material Handling
- ❏ Is there lifting of loads, tools, or parts?
- ❏ Is there lowering of loads, tools, or parts?
- ❏ Is there overhead reaching for loads, tools, or parts?
- ❏ Is there bending at the waist to handle loads, tools, or parts?
- ❏ Is there twisting at the waist to handle loads, tools, or parts?

Physical Energy Demands
- ❏ Do tools and parts weigh more than 10 lbs?
- ❏ Is reaching greater than 20 inches?
- ❏ Is bending, stooping, or squatting a primary task activity?
- ❏ Is lifting or lowering loads a primary task activity?
- ❏ Is walking or carrying loads a primary task activity?
- ❏ Is stair or ladder climbing with loads a primary task activity?
- ❏ Is pushing or pulling loads a primary task activity?
- ❏ Is reaching overhead a primary task activity?
- ❏ Do any of the above tasks require five or more complete work cycles to be done within a minute?
- ❏ Do workers complain that rest breaks and fatigue allowances are insufficient?

Other Musculoskeletal Demands
- ❏ Do manual jobs require frequent, repetitive motions?
- ❏ Do work postures require frequent bending of the neck, shoulder, elbow, wrist, or finger joints?
- ❏ For seated work, do reaches for tools and materials exceed 15 inches from the worker's position?
- ❏ Is the worker unable to change his or her position often?
- ❏ Does the work involve forceful, quick, or sudden motions?
- ❏ Does the work involve shock or rapid buildup of forces?
- ❏ Is finger-pinch gripping used?
- ❏ Do job postures involve sustained muscle contraction of any limb?

Computer Workstation
- ❏ Do operators use computer workstations for more than 4 hours a day?
- ❏ Are there complaints of discomfort from those working at these stations?
- ❏ Is the chair or desk nonadjustable?
- ❏ Is the display monitor, keyboard, or document holder nonadjustable?
- ❏ Does lighting cause glare or make the monitor screen hard to read?
- ❏ Is the room temperature too hot or too cold?
- ❏ Is there irritating vibration or noise?

Environment
- ❏ Is the temperature too hot or too cold?
- ❏ Are the worker's hands exposed to temperatures less than 70° F?
- ❏ Is the workplace poorly lit?
- ❏ Is there glare?
- ❏ Is there excessive noise that is annoying, distracting, or producing hearing loss?
- ❏ Is there upper extremity or whole body vibration?
- ❏ Is air circulation too high or too low?

General Workplace
- ❏ Are walkways uneven, slippery, or obstructed?
- ❏ Is housekeeping poor?
- ❏ Is there inadequate clearance or accessibility for performing tasks?
- ❏ Are stairs cluttered or lacking railings?
- ❏ Is proper footwear worn?

FIGURE 2-15 General ergonomic risk analysis checklist. (From Cohen AL, et al: *Elements of ergonomics programs: A primer based on workplace evaluations of musculoskeletal disorders,* Washington DC, 1997, US Government Printing Office.)

Tools

- ❏ Is the handle too small or too large?
- ❏ Does the handle shape cause the operator to bend the wrist in order to use the tool?
- ❏ Is the tool hard to access?
- ❏ Does the tool weigh more than 9 pounds?
- ❏ Does the tool vibrate excessively?
- ❏ Does the tool cause excessive kickback to the operator?
- ❏ Does the tool become too hot or too cold?

Gloves

- ❏ Do the gloves require the worker to use more force when performing job tasks?
- ❏ Do the gloves provide inadequate protection?
- ❏ Do the gloves present a hazard of catch points on the tool or in the workplace?

Administration

- ❏ Is there little worker control over the work process?
- ❏ Is the task highly repetitive and monotonous?
- ❏ Does the job involve critical tasks with high accountability and little or no tolerance for error?
- ❏ Are work hours and breaks poorly organized?

FIGURE 2-15, cont'd

Risk Analysis Checklist for Computer-User Workstations

"No" responses indicate potential problem areas which should receive further investigation.

1. Does the workstation ensure proper worker posture, such as

   - horizontal thighs? ☐ Yes ☐ No
   - vertical lower legs? ☐ Yes ☐ No
   - feet flat on floor or footrest? ☐ Yes ☐ No
   - neutral wrists? ☐ Yes ☐ No

2. Does the chair

   - adjust easily? ☐ Yes ☐ No
   - have a padded seat with a rounded front? ☐ Yes ☐ No
   - have an adjustable backrest? ☐ Yes ☐ No
   - provide lumbar support? ☐ Yes ☐ No
   - have casters? ☐ Yes ☐ No

3. Are the height and tilt of the work surface on which the keyboard is located adjustable? ☐ Yes ☐ No

4. Is the keyboard detachable? ☐ Yes ☐ No

5. Do keying actions require minimal force? ☐ Yes ☐ No

6. Is there an adjustable document holder? ☐ Yes ☐ No

7. Are arm rests provided where needed? ☐ Yes ☐ No

8. Are glare and reflections avoided? ☐ Yes ☐ No

9. Does the monitor have brightness and contrast controls? ☐ Yes ☐ No

10. Do the operators judge the distance between eyes and work to be satisfactory for their viewing needs? ☐ Yes ☐ No

11. Is there sufficient space for knees and feet? ☐ Yes ☐ No

12. Can the workstation be used for either right- or left-handed activity? ☐ Yes ☐ No

13. Are adequate rest breaks provided for task demands? ☐ Yes ☐ No

14. Are high stroke rates avoided by

    - job rotation? ☐ Yes ☐ No
    - self-pacing? ☐ Yes ☐ No
    - adjusting the job to the skill of the worker? ☐ Yes ☐ No

15. Are employees trained in

    - proper postures? ☐ Yes ☐ No
    - proper work methods? ☐ Yes ☐ No
    - when and how to adjust their workstations? ☐ Yes ☐ No
    - how to seek assistance for their concerns? ☐ Yes ☐ No

FIGURE 2-16 Risk analysis checklist for computer-user workstations. (From Cohen AL, Gjessing CC, Fine LJ, et al: *Elements of ergonomics programs: A primer based on workplace evaluations of musculoskeletal disorders* (DHHS [NIOSH] Publ. No. 97-117). Washington DC, U.S. Government Printing Office, 1997.)

Handtool Risk Factor Checklist

"No" responses indicate potential problem areas which should receive further investigation.

1. Are tools selected to limit or minimize

   - exposure to excessive vibration? ☐ Yes ☐ No
   - use of excessive force? ☐ Yes ☐ No
   - bending or twisting the wrist? ☐ Yes ☐ No
   - finger pinch grip? ☐ Yes ☐ No
   - problems associated with trigger finger? ☐ Yes ☐ No

2. Are tools powered where necessary and feasible? ☐ Yes ☐ No

3. Are tools evenly balanced? ☐ Yes ☐ No

4. Are heavy tools suspended or counterbalanced in ways to facilitate use? ☐ Yes ☐ No

5. Does the tool allow adequate visibility of the work? ☐ Yes ☐ No

6. Does the tool grip/handle prevent slipping during use? ☐ Yes ☐ No

7. Are tools equipped with handles of textured, non-conductive material? ☐ Yes ☐ No

8. Are different handle sizes available to fit a wide range of hand sizes? ☐ Yes ☐ No

9. Is the tool handle designed not to dig in the palm of the hand? ☐ Yes ☐ No

10. Can the tool be used safely with gloves? ☐ Yes ☐ No

11. Can the tool be used by either hand? ☐ Yes ☐ No

12. Is there a preventative maintenance program to keep tools operating as designed? ☐ Yes ☐ No

13. Have employees been trained

   - in the proper use of tools? ☐ Yes ☐ No
   - when and how to report problems with tools? ☐ Yes ☐ No
   - in proper tool maintenance? ☐ Yes ☐ No

FIGURE 2-17 Hand tool risk factor checklist. (From Cohen AL, Gjessing CC, Fine LJ, et al: *Elements of ergonomics programs: A primer based on workplace evaluations of musculoskeletal disorders* (DHHS [NIOSH] Publ. No. 97-117). Washington DC, U.S. Government Printing Office, 1997.)

Americans With Disabilities Act and Related Laws That Promote Participation in Work, Leisure, and Activities of Daily Living

BOX 2-4   Disability Etiquette Dos and Don'ts

- Do try to treat an individual with disabilities as you would treat any other person.
- Don't raise your voice at someone because he or she is in a wheelchair or has a visual or hearing impairment.
- Do address the person, not the wheelchair, interpreter, or guide.
- Don't trap yourself into thinking, "If I were disabled, how would I feel?"
- Do refer to an individual with a disability as "an individual with a disability."
- Don't refer to an individual with a disability as "the quadriplegic," or "Mary is diabetic or epileptic."
- Do cleanse your vocabulary of offensive, outdated terms such as wheelchair-bound or stroke "victim," "afflicted with…," "suffering from…."
- Don't refer to able-bodied persons as "normal."
- Do avoid generalizations such as "people with epilepsy are unpredictable" or "people with learning disabilities are not very intelligent."
- Don't apologize for comments such as "Let's take a walk" to an individual in a wheelchair or "Do you see my point?" to a person with a visual impairment.
- Do avoid statements such as, "I admire your courage" or "You've done so much for a person in a wheelchair."
- Don't use outdated terminology such as "handicapped," "crippled," "retarded," "lame," "the disabled," or "the handicapped."
- Do provide assistance only in the manner requested.
- Don't take hold of an individual's wheelchair or push his or her wheelchair unless asked to do so.
- Do put yourself on the same level as the individual in a wheelchair as soon as possible by sitting down during the conversation or interview.
- Don't turn away when conversing with an individual with a hearing impairment.
- Do speak directly to the person, not the interpreter.
- Don't complete the sentences of an individual with communication impairments.
- Do rid your thinking of stereotypes about disabilities.
- Don't perpetuate another person's insensitivity to an individual with a disability.

Courtesy Barbara L. Kornblau, ADA Consultants, South Miami, Fla.

Leisure Occupations

TABLE 2-5 Leisure Assessments and Descriptions Used by Occupational Therapists

Assessment	Description
Occupational profile	Interview with client (and family, caregivers, if appropriate) to gather information about demographics, language, health status, social and medical history. Questions addressing why client needs OT services, his or her concerns, occupational history (e.g., values, meanings associated with life experiences), and client's priorities
Canadian occupational performance measure	Interview conducted pre- and postintervention to describe problems, level of satisfaction with performing activities, level of perceived performance abilities in areas of self-care, productivity, leisure
Role checklist	Interview to discover past, present, and future occupational roles (including leisure roles) and their value to client
Activity card sort	Picture cards of adults performing instrumental, social-cultural, and leisure activities. Client sorts them into piles depending on interest level. Provides a retained activity level score indicating engagement levels of activity performance of past and current activities.
Modified Interest Checklist (available from Model of Human Occupation Clearinghouse)	Checklist of 68 activity items that assesses client's level of interest (casual, strong, or no interest); includes many leisure time activities
Leisure attitude measurement scale	Scale of 36 items addressing attitudes toward leisure in three areas: cognitive, affective, and behavioral; rated on a five-point scale from "never true" to "always true"
Leisure motivation scale	Scale of 48 items addressing motivation to participate in leisure in four areas: intellectual activities, social activities, mastery activities, and stimulus-avoidance activities; rated on a five-point scale from "never true" to "always true"
Quality of life scale	Perceived quality of life on a scale of 16 items (e.g., material comforts, expressing yourself creatively, socializing, participating in active recreation) rated on a Likert scale of "very satisfied" to "very dissatisfied"
Play and laughter assessment	Informal interview to determine, for example, client's attitude toward humor use, sense of humor, types of humor client has enjoyed
Performance skills	Assessment of client's ability to perform leisure occupations; includes motor skills, process skills, communication, and interaction skills. These may be assessed using formal tests and by observation and analysis of client's performance during activity engagement in the appropriate context (e.g., analyze the client's ability to hold and manipulate cards during a card game; analyze client's ability to put bait on a fish hook, manage the rod and reel, catch and remove fish from hook while seated by a lake).
Ohio Functional Assessment Battery: Standardized tests for leisure and living skills	Designed for use with cognitively impaired individuals; structured interview or questionnaire assessing interests, resources, participation, motivation, and barriers to therapy. Has three test options: functional living skills assessment, quick functional screening test, and recreation and leisure profile.

Continued

TABLE 2-5 Leisure Assessments and Descriptions Used by Occupational Therapists—cont'd

Assessment	Description
Context	Assessment of cultural, physical, social, personal, spiritual, temporal, and virtual contexts that may influence participation in leisure occupations
Client factors	Assessment of body systems that support participation in leisure occupations (e.g., mental, sensory, neuromusculoskeletal, cardiovascular, respiratory and speech functions, pain, skin)

Performance Skills and Client Factors: Evaluation and Intervention

Assistive Technology

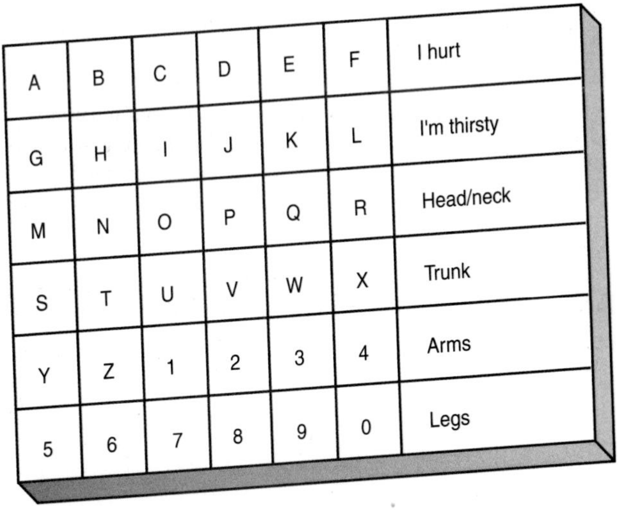

A	B	C	D	E	F	I hurt
G	H	I	J	K	L	I'm thirsty
M	N	O	P	Q	R	Head/neck
S	T	U	V	W	X	Trunk
Y	Z	1	2	3	4	Arms
5	6	7	8	9	0	Legs

FIGURE 3-1 Low-technology augmentative and alternative communication (AAC) system.

Evaluation of Motor Control

Observing movements during occupational performance is a way to assess motor control. Following an evaluation of occupational performance, it may be necessary to evaluate the specific components that underlie motor control. These components are muscle tone, postural tone, and the postural mechanism, reflexes, selective movement, and coordination.

The following questions may be helpful to guide observation of motor control dysfunction.

1. Is the client having difficulty with sitting or standing balance?
2. Is the client having difficulty making appropriate postural adjustments of the trunk and limbs to achieve the best position and motions needed to perform the activity?
3. Is there adequate trunk control to perform the activity?

4. Do changes in body and head position affect muscle tone?
5. Are primitive reflexes evoked during performance?
6. Is there hypertonicity limiting antagonist movement?
7. Are spatial or temporal sequencing problems interfering with coordinated movement?
8. Is there weakness that prohibits antigravity activity?
9. Are tremors, athetoid, or choreiform movements apparent?
10. Is there apparent incoordination (e.g., overshooting or under-shooting the target)? Are there extraneous movements?
11. Describe the spontaneous functional use of the involved extremities.

Assessments for Motor Control Problems

1. The Graded Wolf Motor Function Test (GWMFT) is a new assessment developed to measure functional gains after a hemiparetic event from a cerebrovascular accident (CVA) or traumatic brain injury (TBI). This test was based on the Wolf Motor Function Test. It is called graded because there are two levels of difficulty for each task; level A is more advanced and level B is easier.
2. The Wolf Motor Function Test (WMFT) has been used to quantify the motor abilities of chronic clients from a population of those with high upper extremity function following a CVA or TBI.
3. The Functional Test for the Hemiplegic-Paretic Upper Extremity assesses the client's ability to use the involved arm for purposeful tasks. This test provides objective documentation of functional improvement and includes tasks ranging from those that involve basic stabilization to more difficult tasks requiring fine manipulation and proximal stabilization.
4. The Fugl-Myer assessment is based on the natural progression of neurologic recovery after CVA and is a quantitative assessment of motor function following stroke by measuring such parameters as range of motion (ROM), pain, sensation, and balance.
5. The Arm Motor Ability Test (AMAT) is a functional assessment of upper extremity function. Cutting meat, making a sandwich, opening a jar, and putting on a T-shirt are some of the tasks included in this test.
6. The Motricity Index (MI) is a valid and reliable test of motor impairment that can be performed quickly. The test assesses

pinching a cube with the index finger and thumb, as well as elbow flexion, shoulder abduction, ankle dorsiflexion, knee extension, and hip flexion.

7. The Assessment of Motor and Process Skills (AMPS) is a standardized test that assesses motor and process skills in IADLs. Although the test is not diagnosis-specific, it has been widely used with clients who have had a CVA.

MUSCLE TONE ASSESSMENT

It is important to note the client's overall posture during the evaluation of muscle tone. Is the client's posture symmetrical, with equal weight bearing on both hips (if sitting) or on both feet (if standing)? Note how the client moves in general. Is the head aligned or tilted to one side? Is one shoulder elevated? Is the trunk rotated or elongated on one side and shortened on the other? Such abnormalities will affect the client's ability to move the limbs normally. Current intervention focuses heavily on quality of movement, achieving as normal motor control as possible during occupation.

BOX 3-1 Ashworth Scale

0 = Normal muscle tone
1 = Slight increase in muscle tone, "catch" when limb moved
2 = More marked increase in muscle tone, but limb easily flexed
3 = Considerable increase in muscle tone
4 = Limb rigid in flexion or extension

From Ashworth B: Preliminary trial of carisoprodol in multiple sclerosis. *Practitioner* 192:540-542, 1964.

BOX 3-2 Mild-Moderate-Severe Spasticity Scale

Mild: The stretch reflex (palpable catch) occurs at the muscle's end range (i.e., the muscle is in a lengthened position).
Moderate: The stretch reflex (palpable catch) occurs in midrange.
Severe: The stretch reflex (palpable catch) occurs when the muscle is in a shortened range.

Adapted from Farber S: *Neurorehabilitation: A multisensory approach*, Philadelphia, WB Saunders, 1982.

BOX 3-3 Preston's Hypertonicity Scale

0: No abnormal tone detected during slow, passive movement.
1 or mild: First tone or resistance felt when the muscle is in lengthened position during slow passive movement.
2 or moderate: First tone or resistance felt in midrange of the muscle during slow passive movement
3 or severe: First tone or resistance occurs when the muscle is in shortened range during slow passive movement.

TABLE 3-1 Modified Brunnstrom Stages of Motor Recovery*:

Brunnstrom Stage	Motor Recovery of Arm and Hand	Interdisciplinary Spasticity Management Options
1	Flaccidity. No active movement.	Prevent contractures with PROM and splinting; risk for metacarpophalangeal extension contractures.
2	Beginning development of spasticity, weak synergistic movement of scapular retractors, scapular elevators, elbow flexors, and forearm pronators.	Prevent contractures with PROM and splinting. Risk for shoulder, elbow, forearm, and finger flexion contractures. Promote active movement in gravity-reduced planes. Blocks or surgery are generally not indicated at this stage.
3	Spasticity increasing. Synergy pattern can possibly be useful for carrying objects. Synergy patterns or some of their components can be performed voluntarily. Gross grasp is developing, but no finger release. Lateral pinch possible via thumb adduction tone and flexor pollicis longus tone.	Acute: Good candidate for nerve or motor point blocks† to prevent contractures. There may be a possibility of facilitating recovery by unmasking movement in antagonists if the spastic agonists are weakened through blocks. See text for occupational therapy treatment suggestions. Chronic: After all conservative measures have failed, orthopedic surgery to release contractures to improve hygiene in the hand and ease upper extremity dressing.
4	Spasticity declining; movement combinations from synergies are now possible. Elbow, wrist, and finger extension are emerging but are not to full range.	Acute: Good to excellent nerve block candidate. Better chance of gaining motor control of antagonists with blocks to the spastic agonists. See text for occupational therapy treatment suggestions. Chronic: Ongoing blocks three to four times per year if the risk-benefit ratio for orthopedic surgery is not acceptable to the client. Orthopedic surgery options include procedures to gain function and ameliorate contractures.
5	Synergies are no longer dominant. Emergence of intrinsic function. Finger extension is full range. Isolated finger extension is possible. Three-jaw chuck pinch is possible, but has poor motor control.	Excellent candidate for fine-tuning motor control via blocks (e.g., blocking the extrinsic flexor pollicis longus with the goal of facilitating intrinsic motor control of the thumb, opponens pollicis, abductor pollicis brevis, and flexor pollicis brevis).
6	All types of prehension. Isolated joint movements are perfromed with ease. Intrinsic function is normal.	The client is not a candidate for blocks or surgery. Discharge occupational therapy, as goals were met.

NOTE: Upper extremity recovery is variable because of varying degrees of paralysis. Some clients may never progress through all the stages.

*Guidelines for interdisciplinary spasticity management in subjects with CVA or hemiparesis from TBI.

†Blocks refer to chemical denervation with botulinum toxin type A or B or neurolysis or motor point blocks with phenol or alcohol.

Adapted from Brunnstrom S: *Movement therapy in hemiplegia*. Philadelphia, Lippincott Williams & Wilkins, 1970.

Occupation-Based Functional Motion Assessment

The occupation-based functional motion assessment is a way of assessing ROM, strength, and motor control available for task performance by observing the client during performance of functional occupations (activities of daily living [ADLs], instrumental activities of daily living [IADLs], work, or leisure activities) in varied contexts and environments.

Joint Range of Motion

General Procedure: 180-Degree Method of Measurement

1. The client should be comfortable and relaxed in the appropriate position (see later) for the joint measurement.
2. Uncover the joint to be measured.
3. Explain and demonstrate to the client what you are going to do, why, and how you expect him or her to cooperate.
4. If there is unilateral involvement, assess the PROM on the analogous limb to establish normal ROM for the client.
5. Establish and palpate bony landmarks for the measurement.
6. Stabilize joints proximal to the joint being measured.
7. Move the part passively through ROM to assess joint mobility and end feel.
8. Return the part to the starting position.
9. To measure the starting position, place the goniometer just over the surface of and lateral to the joint.

Place the axis of the goniometer over the axis of the joint, using the designated bony prominence or anatomic landmark. Place the stationary bar on or parallel to the longitudinal axis of the proximal or stationary bone and the movable bar on or parallel to the longitudinal axis of the distal or moving bone. To prevent the indicator on the movable bar from going off the protractor dial, always face the curved side away from the direction of motion, unless the goniometer can be read after movement in either direction.

- Record the number of degrees at the starting position and remove (or back off) the goniometer. Do not attempt to hold the goniometer in place while moving the joint through ROM.

- To measure PROM, hold the part securely above and below the joint being measured and gently move the joint through ROM. Do not force the joints. Watch for signs of pain and discomfort. (**NOTE:** PROM may also be measured by asking the client to move actively through ROM and hold the position. The therapist then moves the joint through the final few degrees of PROM.)
- Reposition the goniometer and record the number of degrees at the final position.
- Remove the goniometer and gently place the part in resting position.
- Record the reading at final position and any notations on the evaluation form.

TABLE 3-2 Average Normal Range of Motion (180-Degree Method)

Joint	Range of Motion (degrees)	Associated Girdle Motion
Cervical Spine		
Flexion	0-45	
Extension	0-45	
Lateral flexion	0-45	
Rotation	0-60	
Thoracic and Lumbar Spine		
Flexion	0-80	
Extension	0-30	
Lateral flexion	0-40	
Rotation	0-45	
Shoulder		
Flexion	0-170	Abduction, lateral tilt, slight elevation, slight upward rotation
Extension	0-60	Depression, adduction, upward tilt
Abduction	0-170	Upward rotation, elevation
Adduction	0	Depression, adduction, downward rotation
Horizontal abduction	0-40	Adduction, reduction of lateral tilt
Horizontal adduction	0-180	Abduction, lateral tilt
Internal rotation		Abduction, lateral tilt
Arm in abduction	0-70	
Arm in adduction	0-40	
External rotation		Adduction, reduction of lateral tilt
Arm in abduction	0-90	
Arm in abduction	0-60	
Elbow		
Flexion	0-135-140	
Extension	0	

Continued

TABLE 3-2 Average Normal Range of Motion (180-Degree Method)—cont'd

Joint	Range of Motion (degrees)	Associated Girdle Motion
Forearm		
Pronation	0-80-90	
Supination	0-80-90	
Wrist		
Flexion	0-80	
Extension	0-70	
Ulnar deviation (adduction)	0-30	
Radial deviation (abduction)	0-20	
Thumb		
DIP Flexion	0 to 80-90	
MP flexion	0-50	
Adduction, radial and palmar	0	
Palmar abduction	0-50	
Radial abduction	0-50	
Opposition		Thumb pad; touch pad of little finger
Fingers		
MP flexion	0-90	
MP hyperextension	0-15-45	
PIP flexion	0-110	
DIP flexion	0-80	
Abduction	0-25	
Hip		
Flexion	0-120 (bent knee)	
Extension	0-30	
Abduction	0-40	
Adduction	0-35	
Internal rotation	0-45	
External rotation	0-45	
Knee		
Flexion	0-135	
Ankle and Foot		
Plantar flexion	0-50	
Dorsiflexion	0-15	
Inversion	0-35	
Eversion	0-20	

DIP, Distal interphalangeal; MP, metacarpophalangeal; PIP, proximal interphalangeal.

Data adapted from American Academy of Orthopaedic Surgeons: *Joint Motion: Method of measuring and Recording,* Chicago, American Academy of Orthopaedic Surgeons, 1965; Esch D, Lepley M: *Evaluation of joint motion: methods of measurement and recording,* Minneapolis, University of Minnesota Press, 1974.

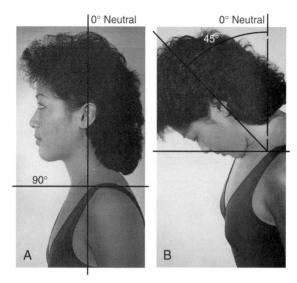

FIGURE 3-2 Cervical flexion. **A,** Starting position. **B,** Final position.

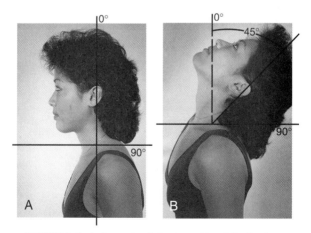

FIGURE 3-3 Cervical extension. **A,** Starting position. **B,** Final position.

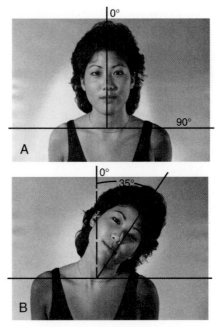

FIGURE 3-4 Cervical lateral flexion. **A,** Starting position. **B,** Final position.

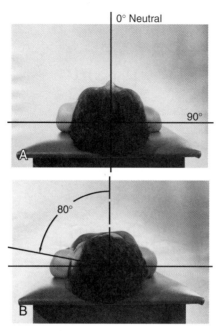

FIGURE 3-5 Cervical rotation. **A,** Starting position. **B,** Final position.

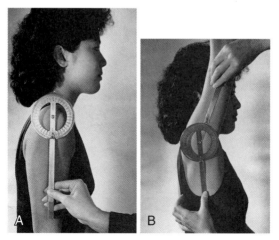

FIGURE 3-6 Shoulder flexion. **A,** Starting position. **B,** Final position.

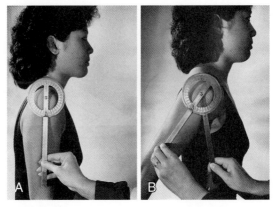

FIGURE 3-7 Shoulder extension. **A,** Starting position. **B,** Final position.

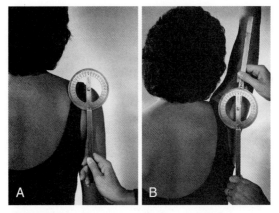

FIGURE 3-8 Shoulder abduction. **A,** Starting position. **B,** Final position.

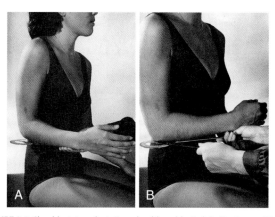

FIGURE 3-9 Shoulder internal rotation, shoulder adducted. **A,** Starting position. **B,** Final position.

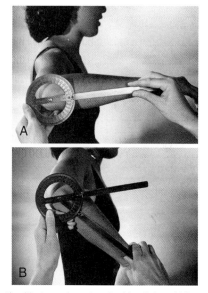

FIGURE 3-10 Shoulder internal rotation, shoulder abducted (alternative position). **A,** Starting position. **B,** Final position.

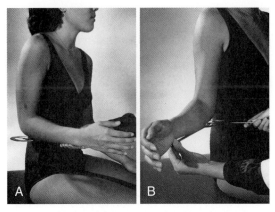

FIGURE 3-11 Shoulder external rotation, shoulder adducted. **A,** Starting position. **B,** Final position.

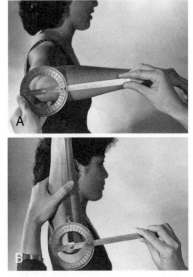

FIGURE 3-12 Shoulder external rotation, shoulder abducted (alternative position). **A,** Starting position. **B,** Final position.

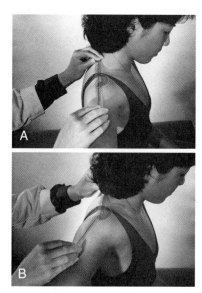

FIGURE 3-13 Shoulder horizontal abduction. **A,** Starting position. **B,** Final position.

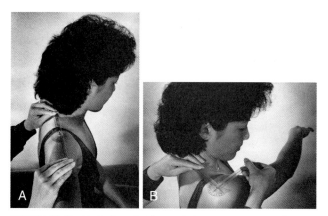

FIGURE 3-14 Shoulder horizontal adduction. **A,** Starting position. **B,** Final position.

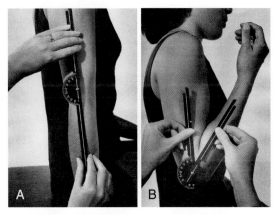

FIGURE 3-15 Elbow flexion. **A,** Starting position. **B,** Final position.

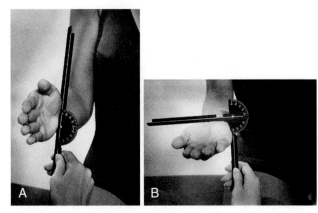

FIGURE 3-16 Forearm supination. **A,** Starting position. **B,** Final position.

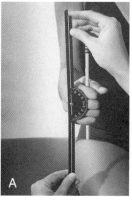
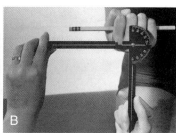

FIGURE 3-17 Forearm supination (alternate method). **A,** Starting position. **B,** Final position.

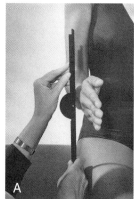
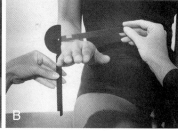

FIGURE 3-18 Forearm pronation. **A,** Starting position. **B,** Final position.

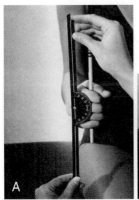
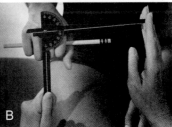

FIGURE 3-19 Forearm pronation (alternate method). **A,** Starting position. **B,** Final position.

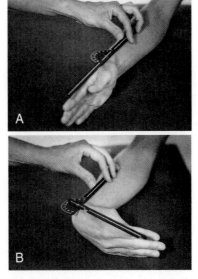

FIGURE 3-20 Wrist flexion. **A,** Starting position. **B,** Final position.

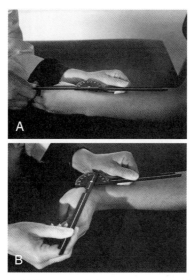

FIGURE 3-21 Wrist extension. **A,** Starting position. **B,** Final position.

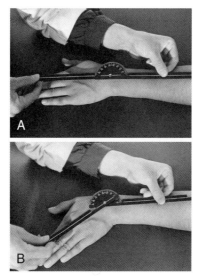

FIGURE 3-22 Wrist ulnar deviation. **A,** Starting position. **B,** Final position.

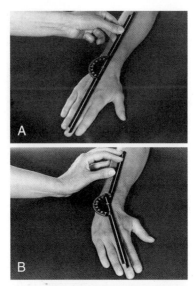

FIGURE 3-23 Wrist radial deviation. **A,** Starting position. **B,** Final position.

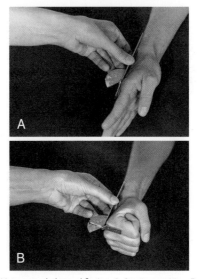

FIGURE 3-24 Metacarpophalangeal flexion. **A,** Starting position. **B,** Final position.

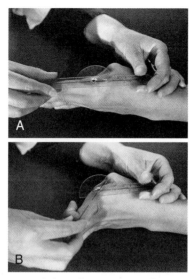

FIGURE 3-25 Metacarpophalangeal hyperextension. **A,** Starting position. **B,** Final position.

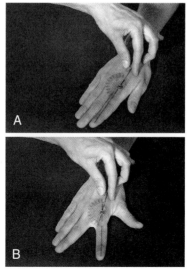

FIGURE 3-26 Metacarpophalangeal abduction. **A,** Starting position. **B,** Final position.

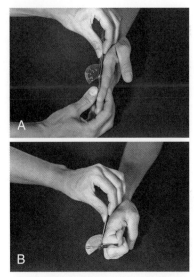

FIGURE 3-27 Proximal interphalangeal flexion. **A,** Starting position. **B,** Final position.

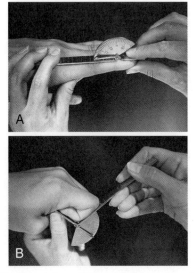

FIGURE 3-28 Distal interphalangeal flexion. **A,** Starting position. **B,** Final position.

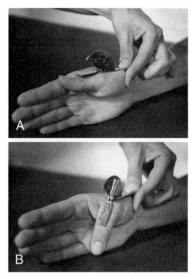

FIGURE 3-29 Thumb metacarpophalangeal flexion. **A,** Starting position. **B,** Final position.

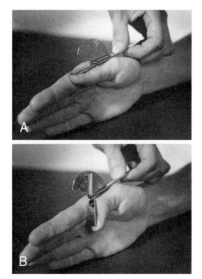

FIGURE 3-30 Thumb interphalangeal flexion. **A,** Starting position. **B,** Final position.

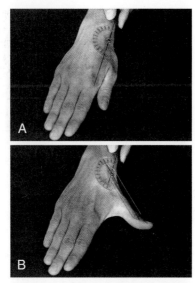

FIGURE 3-31 Thumb radial abduction. **A,** Starting position. **B,** Final position.

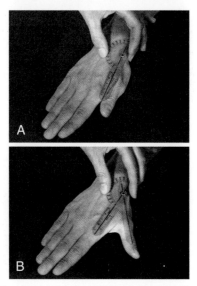

FIGURE 3-32 Thumb radial abduction (alternative method). **A,** Starting position. **B,** Final position.

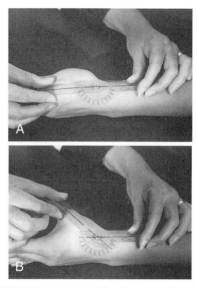

FIGURE 3-33 Palmar abduction. **A,** Starting position. **B,** Final position.

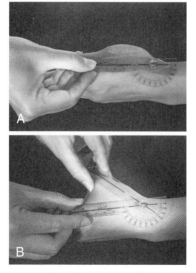

FIGURE 3-34 Palmar abduction (alternative method). **A,** Starting position. **B,** Final position.

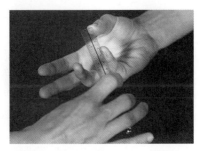

FIGURE 3-35 Thumb opposition to fifth finger.

Evaluation of Muscle Strength

A loss of muscle strength is a primary symptom or a direct result of the following diseases or injuries:

1. Lower motor neuron disorders, such as peripheral neuropathies and peripheral nerve injuries, spinal cord injury (because those muscles innervated at the level[s] of the lesion generally have a lower motor neuron paralysis), Guillain-Barré syndrome, and cranial nerve dysfunctions
2. Primary muscle diseases, such as muscular dystrophy and myasthenia gravis
3. Neurologic diseases in which the lower motor neuron is affected, such as amyotrophic lateral sclerosis or multiple sclerosis

The manual muscle test (MMT) is a means of evaluating muscle strength. MMT measures the maximal contraction of a muscle or muscle group. The criteria used to measure strength are evidence of muscle contraction, amount of ROM through which the joint passes when the muscle contracts, and amount of resistance against which the muscle can contract. Gravity is considered a form of resistance.

Contraindications

Assessment of strength using MMT is contraindicated when the client has inflammation or pain in the region to be tested, a dislocation or unhealed fracture, recent surgery, particularly of musculoskeletal structures, myositis ossificans, or bone carcinoma or any fragile bone condition.

TABLE 3-3 Muscle Grades and Their Definitions

Number Grade	Word or Letter Grade	Definition
0	Zero (0)	No muscle contraction can be seen or felt.
1	Trace (T)	Contraction can be observed or felt, but there is no motion.
2−	Poor minus (P−)	Part moves through incomplete ROM with gravity minimized.
2	Poor (P)	Part moves through complete ROM with gravity minimized.
2+	Poor plus (P+)	Part moves through less than 50% of available ROM against gravity or through complete ROM with gravity minimized against slight resistance.
3−	Fair minus (F−)	Part moves through more than 50% of available ROM against gravity.
3	Fair (F)	Part moves through complete ROM against gravity.
3+	Fair plus (F+)	Part moves through complete ROM against gravity and slight resistance.
4	Good (G)	Part moves through complete ROM against gravity and moderate resistance.
5	Normal (N)	Part moves through complete ROM against gravity and maximal resistance.

Manual Muscle Testing of the Upper Extremity: Scapula Elevation, Neck Rotation, and Lateral Flexion

Muscles	Innervation: nerve, nerve roots
Upper trapezius	Accessory nerve (CN 12), C2-4
Levator scapula	Dorsal scapular nerve, C3-5

PROCEDURE FOR TESTING GRADES NORMAL (N OR 5) TO FAIR (F OR 3)

1. Position: The client is seated erect with arms resting at sides of body. The occupational therapist (OT) practitioner stands behind the client toward the side to be tested.
2. Stabilize: A chair back can offer stabilization to the trunk, if necessary.
3. Palpate: Palpate the upper trapezius parallel to the cervical vertebrae, near the shoulder-neck curve.
4. Observe: Observe the elevation of the scapula as the client shrugs the shoulder toward the ear and rotates and laterally flexes the neck toward the side being tested at the same time.

5. Resist: Provide resistance by placing one hand on top of the shoulder toward the scapular depression and the other hand on the side of the head toward derotation and lateral flexion to the opposite side.

PROCEDURE FOR TESTING GRADES POOR (P OR 2), TRACE (T OR 1), AND ZERO (0)

1. Position: The client should be prone with head in midposition. The OT practitioner stands opposite the side being tested.
2. Stabilize: The weight of the trunk on the supporting surface provides adequate stabilization.
3. Palpate: Palpate the upper trapezius, as described in the previous procedure, while observing the client elevating the shoulder being tested. Because of the positioning, the neck rotation and lateral flexion components are omitted for these grades.
4. Grade: The standard definitions of muscle grades should be used.

Substitutions
Rhomboids and the levator scapula can elevate the scapula if the upper trapezius is weak or absent. In the event of substitution, some downward rotation of the acromion will be observed during the movement.

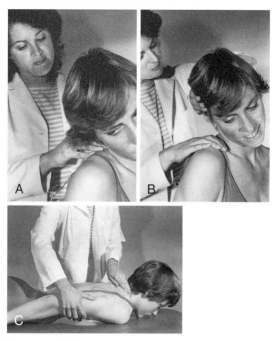

FIGURE 3-36 Scapula elevation. **A,** Palpate and observe. **B,** Resist. **C,** Gravity-minimized position.

Scapula Depression, Adduction, and Upward Rotation

Muscles	Innervation
Lower trapezius	Spinal accessory nerve, C3,4
Middle trapezius	
Serratus anterior	Long thoracic nerve, C5-7

PROCEDURE FOR TESTING GRADES N (5) TO F (3)

1. Position: The client is prone with arm positioned overhead in 130 to 165 degrees of abduction and resting on the supporting surface. The forearm is in midposition with the thumb toward the ceiling. The therapist stands next to the client on the opposite side or on the same side.

2. Stabilize: The weight of the body provides adequate stabilization. This test is given in the gravity-minimized position, because it is not feasible to position the client for the against-gravity movement (head down). If the deltoid is weak, the arm may be supported and passively raised by the therapist while the client attempts the motion.

3. Palpate: Palpate the lower trapezius distal to the medial end of the spine of the scapula and parallel to the thoracic vertebrae, approximately at the level of the inferior angle of the scapula.

4. Observe: Observe the client while he or she lifts the arm off the supporting surface to ear level. During this movement, there is strong downward fixation of the scapula by the lower trapezius.

5. Resist: Provide resistance at the lateral angle of the scapula, toward elevation and abduction. Resistance may be applied on the humerus just above the elbow in a downward direction if shoulder and elbow strength are adequate.

PROCEDURE FOR TESTING GRADES P (2), T (1), AND 0

1. Position and stabilize: Position and stabilize the client as described in the previous test. No stabilization is required. The therapist may support the client's arm if the posterior deltoid muscles and triceps are weak.

2. Palpate and observe: Palpate and observe the client in the same manner as described for the previous test.

3. Grade: The client receives a grade of P if he or she can complete full scapular ROM without the weight of the arm.

Substitutions

The middle trapezius or rhomboids may substitute. Rotation of the inferior angle of the scapula toward the spine is evidence of substitution.

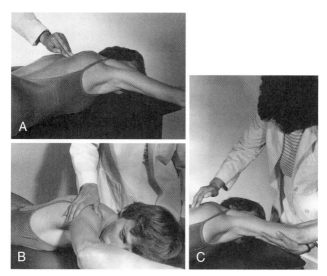

FIGURE 3-37 Scapula depression. **A,** Palpate and observe. **B,** Resist. **C,** Test for grades P to O.

Scapula Abduction and Upward Rotation

Muscles
Serratus anterior

Innervation
Long thoracic nerve, C5-7

PROCEDURE FOR TESTING GRADES N (5) TO F (3)

1. Position: The client is supine with the shoulder flexed to 90 degrees and slightly abducted, elbow extended or fully flexed. The therapist stands next to the client on the side being tested.
2. Stabilize: Provide stabilization over the weight of the trunk or over the shoulder.
3. Palpate: Palpate the digitations of the origin of the serratus anterior on the ribs, along the midaxillary line and just distal and anterior to the axillary border of the scapula. Note that muscle contraction may be difficult to detect in women and overweight clients.
4. Observe: Observe the client reaching upward as if pushing the arm toward the ceiling, abducting the scapula.

5. Resist: Provide resistance at the distal end of the humerus, and push the client's arm directly downward toward scapula adduction. If there is shoulder instability, the therapist should support the arm and not apply resistance. In this case, only a grade of F (3) can be tested.

PROCEDURE FOR TESTING GRADES P (2), T (1), AND O

1. Position: The client is seated with the arm supported by the therapist in 90 degrees of shoulder flexion and the elbow extended.
2. Stabilize: Provide stabilization over the shoulder to be tested.
3. Palpate: The client is palpated in the same manner as described in the previous section.
4. Observe: The therapist should note any abduction of the scapula as the arm moves forward. Weakness of this muscle produces "winging" of the scapula.
5. Grade: The client is graded according to the standard definitions of muscle grades.

Substitutions

The pectoralis major and minor may pull the scapula forward into abduction at its insertion on the humerus; the upper and lower trapezius and contralateral trunk rotation may also substitute. The therapist observes for humeral horizontal adduction followed by scapula abduction.

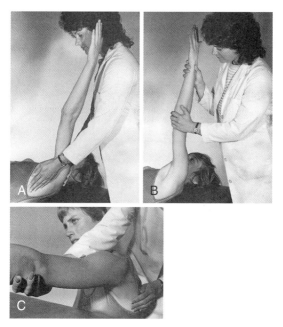

FIGURE 3-38 Scapula abduction. **A,** Palpate and observe. **B,** Resist. **C,** Gravity-minimized position.

Scapula Adduction

Muscles   **Innervation**
Middle trapezius   Spinal accessory nerve, C3,4
Rhomboids   Dorsal scapular nerve, C4,5

PROCEDURE FOR TESTING GRADES N (5) TO F (3)

1. Position: The client is prone with the shoulder abducted to 90 degrees and externally rotated and the elbow flexed to 90 degrees, shoulder resting on the supporting surface. The therapist stands on the side being tested.
2. Stabilize: The weight of the trunk on the supporting surface usually provides adequate stabilization, or stabilization can be provided over the midthorax to prevent trunk rotation if necessary.

3. Palpate: Palpate the middle trapezius between the spine of the scapula and the adjacent vertebrae in alignment with the abducted humerus.
4. Observe: Observe the client lifting the arm off the table, and note any movement of the vertebral border of the scapula toward the thoracic vertebrae.
5. Resist: Provide resistance at the vertebral border of the scapula toward abduction.

PROCEDURE FOR TESTING GRADES P (2), T (1), AND 0

1. Position and stabilize: The therapist positions and stabilizes the client in the same way as described in the previous test but now supports the weight of the arm by cradling it under the humerus and forearm. The client may also be positioned sitting erect, with arm resting on a high table and the shoulder midway between 90-degree flexion and abduction. The therapist stands behind the client In this case.
2. Palpate and observe: Palpate and observe the middle trapezius. Ask the client to bring the shoulders together as if assuming an erect posture. Observe scapula adduction toward the vertebral column.
3. Grade: The client is graded according to the standard definitions of muscle grades.

Substitutions

The posterior deltoid can act on the humerus and produce scapula adduction. Observe for humeral extension being used to initiate scapula adduction. Rhomboids may substitute, but scapula will rotate downward.

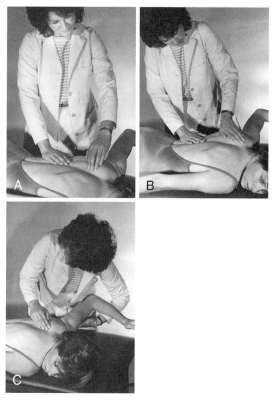

FIGURE 3-39 Scapula adduction. **A,** Palpate and observe. **B,** Resist. **C,** Test for grades P to O.

Scapula Adduction and Downward Rotation

Muscles	Innervation
Rhomboids major and minor	Dorsal scapular nerve, C4,5
Levator scapula	
Middle trapezius	Spinal accessory nerve, C3,4

PROCEDURE FOR TESTING GRADES N (5) TO F (3)

1. Position: The client is prone with the head rotated to the opposite side; the arm on the side being tested is placed in shoulder

adduction and internal rotation, with the elbow slightly flexed and the dorsum of the hand resting over the lumbosacral area of the back. The therapist stands opposite the side being tested.

2. Stabilize: The weight of the trunk on the supporting surface offers adequate stabilization.

3. Palpate: Palpate the rhomboid muscles between the vertebral border of the scapula and the second to fifth thoracic vertebrae. (They may be more easily discerned toward the lower half of the vertebral border of the scapula, because they lie under the trapezius muscle.)

4. Observe: Observe the client raising the hand up off the back while maintaining the position of the arm. During this motion, the anterior aspect of the shoulder must lift from the table surface. Observe scapula adduction and downward rotation while the shoulder joint is in some extension.

5. Resist: Provide resistance over the scapula toward abduction and upward rotation.

PROCEDURE FOR TESTING GRADES P (2), T (1), AND 0

1. Position: The client sits erect with the arm positioned behind the back in the same manner described for the previous test. The therapist stands behind the client, slightly opposite to the side being tested.

2. Stabilize: The trunk is stabilized by placing one hand over the shoulder, opposite the one being tested, to prevent trunk flexion and rotation.

3. Palpate: The rhomboids are palpated as described previously.

4. Observe: Scapula adduction and downward rotation are observed as the client lifts the hand away from the back.

5. Grade: The client is graded according to the standard definitions of muscle grades.

Substitutions

The middle trapezius may substitute, but the movement will not be accompanied by downward rotation. The posterior deltoid acting to perform horizontal abduction or glenohumeral extension can produce scapula adduction through momentum. Scapula adduction would be preceded by extension or abduction of the humerus. The pectoralis minor could tip the scapula forward.

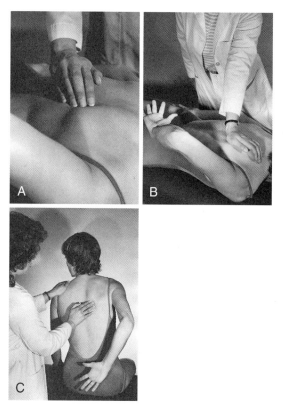

FIGURE 3-40 Scapula adduction and downward rotation. **A,** Palpate and observe. **B,** Resist. **C,** Gravity-minimized position.

Shoulder Flexion

Muscles	Innervation
Anterior deltoid	Axillary nerve, C5,6
Coracobrachialis	Musculocutaneous nerve, C5-7

PROCEDURE FOR TESTING GRADES N (5) TO F (3)

1. Position: The client is seated with the arm relaxed at the side of the body and the hand facing backward. A straight-backed chair

may be used to offer trunk support. The therapist stands on the side being tested and slightly behind the client.

2. Stabilize: Provide stabilization over the shoulder being tested, but allow the normal abduction and upward rotation of the scapula that occurs with this movement.
3. Palpate: Palpate the anterior deltoid just below the clavicle on the anterior aspect of the humeral head.
4. Observe: Observe the client flexing the shoulder joint to 90-degree flexion (parallel to the floor).
5. Resist: Provide resistance at the distal end of the humerus downward toward shoulder extension.

PROCEDURE FOR TESTING GRADES P (2), T (1), AND 0

1. Position: The client is placed in a side-lying position. The side being tested is superior. If the client cannot maintain weight of the arm against gravity, the therapist can support it. If the side-lying position is not feasible, the client may remain seated, and the test procedure described above can be performed with the grading modified.
2. Palpate and observe: The therapist should palpate and observe the client in the same manner as described in the previous test. The arm is moved toward the face to 90-degree shoulder flexion.
3. Grade: The client is graded according to the standard definitions of muscle grades. If the seated position was used for the tests of grades poor to zero, partial ROM against gravity should be graded poor.

Substitutions

Clavicular fibers of the pectoralis major can perform flexion through partial ROM while performing horizontal adduction. The biceps brachii may flex the shoulder, but the humerus will first be rotated externally for the best mechanical advantage. The upper trapezius will assist flexion by elevating the scapula. Observe for flexion accompanied by horizontal adduction, external rotation, or scapula elevation.

Note: Arm elevation in the plane of the scapula, about halfway between shoulder flexion and abduction, is called scaption. This movement is more commonly used for function than shoulder flexion or abduction. Scaption is performed by the deltoid and supraspinatus muscles. It is tested in a way similar to that used for shoulder flexion, described earlier, except that the arm is elevated in a position 30 to 45 degrees anterior to the frontal plane.

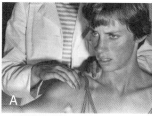
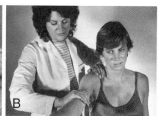
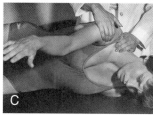

FIGURE 3-41 Shoulder flexion. **A,** Palpate and observe. **B,** Resist. **C,** Gravity-minimized position.

Shoulder Extension

Muscles	Innervation
Latissimus dorsi	Thoracodorsal nerve, C6-8
Teres major	Lower subscapular nerve, C5-7
Posterior deltoid	Axillary nerve, C5,6

PROCEDURE FOR TESTING GRADES N (5) TO F (3)

1. Position: The client is prone, with the shoulder joint adducted and internally rotated so that the palm of the hand is facing up. The therapist stands on the opposite side or on the test side.
2. Stabilize: Provide stabilization over the scapula on the side being tested.
3. Palpate: Palpate the teres major along the axillary border of the scapula. The latissimus dorsi may be palpated slightly below this point or closer to its origins parallel to the thoracic and lumbar vertebrae. The posterior deltoid may be found over the posterior aspect of the humeral head.
4. Observe: Observe the client extending the shoulder joint.

5. Resist: Provide resistance at the distal end of the humerus in a downward and outward direction, toward flexion and slight abduction.

PROCEDURE FOR TESTING GRADES P (2), T (1), AND 0

1. Position: The client is placed in the side-lying position; the therapist stands behind the client.
2. Stabilize: Provide stabilization over the scapula. If the client cannot maintain the weight of the part against gravity, the therapist should support the client's arm. If the side-lying position is not feasible, the client may remain in the prone position and the test may be performed as described for the previous test with modified grading.
3. Palpate: Palpate the teres major or latissimus dorsi as described for the previous test.
4. Observe: Observe the client extending the arm backward in a plane parallel to the floor.
5. Grade: Grade the client according to the standard definitions of muscle grades. If the tests for grades poor to zero was done in the prone-lying position, completion of partial ROM should be graded poor.

Substitutions

Scapula adduction can substitute. Observe for flexion of the shoulder or adduction of the scapula preceding extension of the humerus.

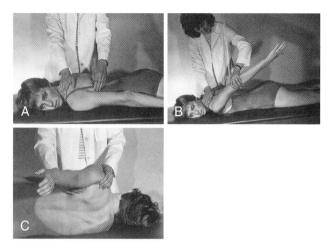

FIGURE 3-42 Shoulder extension. **A,** Palpate and observe. **B,** Resist. **C,** Gravity-minimized position.

Shoulder Abduction to 90 Degrees

Muscles	Innervation
Middle deltoid	Axillary nerve, C5,6
Supraspinatus	Suprascapular nerve, C5

PROCEDURE FOR TESTING GRADES N (5) TO F (3)

1. Position: The client is seated, with arms relaxed at the sides of the body. The elbow on the side to be tested should be slightly flexed and the palms facing toward the body. The therapist stands behind the client.

2. Stabilize: Provide stabilization over the scapula on the side to be tested.

3. Palpate: Palpate the middle deltoid over the middle of the shoulder joint from the acromion to the deltoid tuberosity. The supraspinatus is too deep to palpate.

4. Observe: Observe the client abducting the shoulder to 90 degrees. During the movement, the client's palm should remain down and the therapist should observe that there is no external rotation of the shoulder or elevation of the scapula.

5. Resist: Provide resistance at the distal end of the humerus toward adduction.

PROCEDURE FOR TESTING GRADES P (2), T (1), AND 0

1. Position: The client is in the supine position, lying with the arm to be tested resting at the side of the body, palm facing in and the elbow slightly flexed. The therapist stands in front of the supporting surface toward the side to be tested.
2. Stabilize: Provide stabilization over the shoulder to be tested.
3. Palpate and observe: Follow the technique described for the previous test. The therapist asks the client to bring the arm out and away from the body, abducting the shoulder to 90 degrees.
4. Grade: The client is graded according to the standard definitions of muscle grades.

Substitutions

The long head of the biceps may attempt to substitute. Observe for elbow flexion and external rotation accompanying the movement. The anterior and posterior deltoids can act together to effect abduction. The upper trapezius may attempt to assist. Observe for scapula elevation preceding the movement.

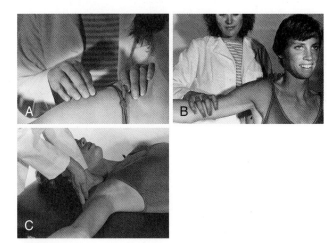

FIGURE 3-43 Shoulder abduction. **A,** Palpate and observe. **B,** Resist. **C,** Gravity-minimized position.

Shoulder External Rotation

Muscles   **Innervation**
Infraspinatus   Suprascapular nerve, C5,6
Teres minor   Axillary nerve, C5,6

PROCEDURE FOR TESTING GRADES N (5) TO F (3)

1. Position: The client is prone, with the shoulder abducted to 90 degrees and the humerus in neutral (0-degree) rotation, elbow flexed to 90 degrees. The forearm is in neutral rotation, hanging over the edge of the table, perpendicular to the floor. The therapist stands in front of the supporting surface, toward the side to be tested.
2. Stabilize: Provide stabilization at the distal end of the humerus by placing a hand under the arm on the supporting surface to prevent shoulder abduction.
3. Palpate: Palpate the infraspinatus muscle just below the spine of the scapula on the body of the scapula or the teres minor along the axillary border of the scapula.
4. Observe: Observe the client rotating the humerus so that the back of the hand is moving toward the ceiling.
5. Resist: Provide resistance on the distal end of the forearm toward the floor in the direction of internal rotation. Apply resistance gently and slowly to prevent injury to the glenohumeral joint, which is inherently unstable.

PROCEDURE FOR TESTING GRADES P (2), T (1), AND 0

1. Position: The client is seated, with arm adducted and in neutral rotation at the shoulder. The elbow is flexed to 90 degrees, with the forearm in neutral rotation. The therapist stands in front of the client toward the side to be tested.
2. Stabilize: Provide stabilization on the arm against the trunk at the distal end of the humerus to prevent abduction and extension of the shoulder, and over the shoulder to be tested. The hand stabilizing over the shoulder can be used to palpate the infraspinatus simultaneously.
3. Palpate: Palpate the infraspinatus and teres minor as described for the previous test.

4. Observe: Observe the client moving the forearm away from the body by rotating the humerus while maintaining neutral rotation of the forearm.
5. Grade: The client is graded according to the standard definitions of muscle grades.

Substitutions

If the elbow is extended and the client supinates the forearm, the momentum could aid external rotation of the humerus. Scapular adduction can pull the humerus backward and into some external rotation. The therapist should observe for scapula adduction and initiation of movement with forearm supination.

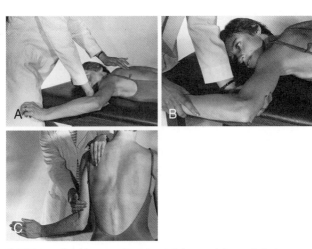

FIGURE 3-44 Shoulder external rotation. **A,** Palpate and observe. **B,** Resist. **C,** Gravity-minimized position.

Shoulder Internal Rotation

Muscles	Innervation
Subscapularis	Subscapular nerve, C5,6
Pectoralis major	Medial and lateral pectoral nerves, C5-T1
Latissimus dorsi	Thoracodorsal nerve, C6-8
Teres major	Subscapular nerve, C5-7

PROCEDURE FOR TESTING GRADES N (5) TO F (3)

1. Position: The client is prone, with the shoulder abducted to 90 degrees, the humerus in neutral rotation, and the elbow flexed to 90 degrees. A rolled towel may be placed under the humerus. The forearm is perpendicular to the floor. The therapist stands on the side to be tested, just in front of the client's arm.
2. Stabilize: Provide stabilization at the distal end of the humerus by placing a hand under the arm and on the supporting surface, as for external rotation.
3. Palpate: Palpate the teres major and latissimus dorsi along the axillary border of the scapula toward the inferior angle.
4. Observe: Observe the client internally rotating the humerus, moving the palm of the hand upward toward the ceiling.
5. Resist: Provide resistance at the distal end of the volar surface of the forearm anteriorly toward external rotation.

PROCEDURE FOR TESTING GRADES P (2), T (1), AND 0

1. Position: The client is seated, with the shoulder adducted and in neutral rotation, elbow flexed to 90 degrees with the forearm in neutral rotation. The therapist stands on the side to be tested.
2. Stabilize: Provide stabilization on the arm at the distal end of the humerus against the trunk to prevent abduction and extension of the shoulder.
3. Palpate: Palpate the teres major and latissimus dorsi, as described for the previous test.
4. Observe: Observe the client moving the palm of the hand toward the chest, internally rotating the humerus.

Substitutions

If the trunk is rotated, gravity will act on the humerus, rotating it internally. The therapist should observe for trunk rotation. When the elbow is in extension, pronation of the forearm can substitute.

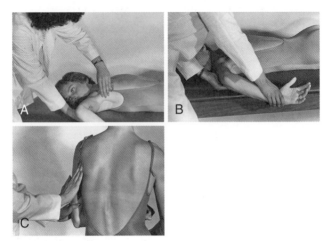

FIGURE 3-45 Shoulder internal rotation. **A,** Palpate and observe. **B,** Resist. **C,** Gravity-minimized position.

Shoulder Horizontal Abduction

Muscles	Innervation
Posterior deltoid	Axillary nerve, C5,6
Infraspinatus	Suprascapular nerve, C5,6

PROCEDURE FOR TESTING GRADES N (5) TO F (3)

1. Position: The client is prone, with the shoulder abducted to 90 degrees and in slight external rotation, elbow flexed to 90 degrees, and forearm perpendicular to the floor. The therapist stands on the side being tested.
2. Stabilize: Provide stabilization over the scapula.
3. Palpate: Palpate the posterior deltoid below the spine of the scapula and distally toward the deltoid tuberosity on the posterior aspect of the shoulder.
4. Observe: Observe the client horizontally abducting the humerus, lifting the arm toward the ceiling.
5. Resist: Provide resistance just proximal to the elbow obliquely downward toward horizontal adduction.

PROCEDURE FOR TESTING GRADES P (2), T (1), AND 0

1. Position: The client is seated, with the arm in 90-degree abduction, the elbow flexed to 90 degrees, and the palm down, supported on a high table or by the therapist. If a table is used, powder may be sprinkled on the surface to reduce friction.
2. Stabilize: Provide stabilization over the scapula.
3. Palpate: Palpate the posterior deltoid, as described for the previous test.
4. Observe: Observe client pulling arm backward into horizontal abduction.
5. Grade: Client is graded according to the standard definitions of muscle grades.

Substitutions

Latissimus dorsi and teres major may assist the movement if the posterior deltoid is very weak. Movement will occur with more shoulder extension rather than at the horizontal level. Scapula adduction may produce slight horizontal abduction of the humerus, but trunk rotation and shoulder retraction would occur. The long head of the triceps may substitute. Maintain some flexion at the elbow to prevent this.

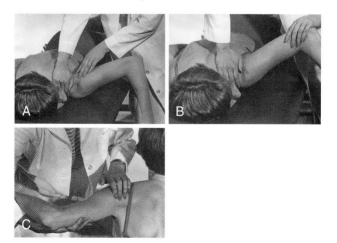

FIGURE 3-46 Shoulder horizontal abduction. **A,** Palpate and observe. **B,** Resist. **C,** Gravity-minimized position.

Shoulder Horizontal Adduction

Muscles   **Innervation**
Pectoralis major   Medial and lateral pectoral nerves, C5-T1
Anterior deltoid   Axillary nerve, C5,6
Coracobrachialis   Musculocutaneous nerve, C6,7

PROCEDURE FOR TESTING GRADES N (5) TO F (3)

1. Position: The client is supine, with the shoulder abducted to 90 degrees, elbow flexed or extended. The therapist stands next to the client on the side being tested or behind C's head.
2. Stabilize: Stabilize the trunk by placing one hand over the shoulder on the side being tested to prevent trunk rotation and scapula elevation.
3. Palpate: Palpate over the insertion of the pectoralis major at the anterior aspect of the axilla.
4. Observe: Observe the client horizontally adducting the humerus, moving the arm toward the opposite shoulder to a position of 90 degrees of shoulder flexion. If the client cannot maintain elbow extension, the therapist may guide the forearm to prevent the hand from hitting the client's face.
5. Resist: Provide resistance at the distal end of the humerus, in an outward direction toward horizontal abduction.

PROCEDURE FOR TESTING GRADES P (2), T (1), AND 0

1. Position: The client is seated next to a high table, with the arm supported in 90 degrees of shoulder abduction and slight flexion at the elbow. Powder may be sprinkled on the supporting surface to reduce the effect of resistance from friction during the movement, or the therapist may support the arm.
2. Stabilize: Provide stabilization over the shoulder on the side being tested, simultaneously using the stabilizing hand to palpate the pectoralis major muscle.
3. Palpate: Palpate the pectoralis major, as described for the previous test.
4. Observe: Observe the client horizontally adducting the arm toward the opposite shoulder, in a plane parallel to the floor.

Substitutions

Muscles may substitute for one another. If the pectoralis major is not functioning, the other muscles will perform the motion, which will be considerably weakened. Contralateral trunk rotation, the coracobrachialis, or the short head of the biceps may substitute.

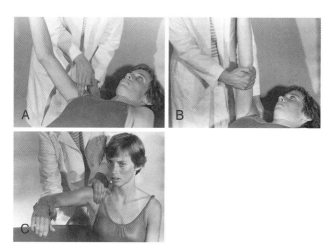

FIGURE 3-47 Shoulder horizontal adduction. **A,** Palpate and observe. **B,** Resist. **C,** Gravity-minimized position.

Elbow Flexion

Muscles	Innervation
Biceps brachii	Musculocutaneous nerve C5,6
Brachialis	
Brachioradialis	Radial nerve C5,6

PROCEDURE FOR TESTING GRADES N (5) TO F (3)

1. Position: The client is seated, with the arm adducted at the shoulder and extended at the elbow and held against the side of the trunk. The forearm is supinated to test for the biceps,

primarily (forearm should be positioned in pronation to test for the brachialis, primarily, and in midposition to test for brachioradialis). The therapist stands next to the client on the side being tested or directly in front of the client.

2. Stabilize: Provide stabilization at the humerus (in adduction).

3. Palpate: Palpate the biceps brachii over the muscle belly, on the middle of the anterior aspect of the humerus. Its tendon may be palpated in the middle of the antecubital space. (Brachioradialis is palpated over the upper third of the radius on the lateral aspect of the forearm, just below the elbow. The brachialis may be palpated lateral to the lower portion of the biceps brachii if the elbow is flexed and in the pronated position.)

4. Observe: Observe the client flexing the elbow, hand toward the face. The therapist should observe for maintenance of forearm in supination (when testing for biceps) and for relaxed or extended wrist and fingers.

5. Resist: Provide resistance at the distal end of the volar aspect of the forearm, pulling downward toward elbow extension.

PROCEDURE FOR TESTING GRADES P (2), T (1), AND 0

1. Position: The client is supine, with the shoulder abducted to 90 degrees and externally rotated, elbow extended, and forearm supinated. The therapist stands at the head of the table on the side being tested. (The client may also be seated, side being tested resting on the treatment table, which is at axillary height, humerus in 90-degree abduction, elbow extended, and forearm in neutral position.)

2. Stabilize: Provide stabilization at the humerus. The stabilizing hand can be used simultaneously for palpation here.

3. Palpate: Palpate the biceps as described for the previous test.

4. Observe: Observe the client flexing the elbow, with the hand toward the shoulder. Watch for maintenance of forearm supination and relaxation of the fingers and wrist.

5. Grade: The client is graded according to the standard definitions of muscle grades.

Substitutions

The brachioradialis will substitute for the biceps, but the forearm will move to midposition during flexion of the elbow. Wrist and finger flexors may assist elbow flexion, which will be preceded by finger and wrist flexion. The pronator teres may assist. Forearm pronation during the movement may be evidence of this substitution.

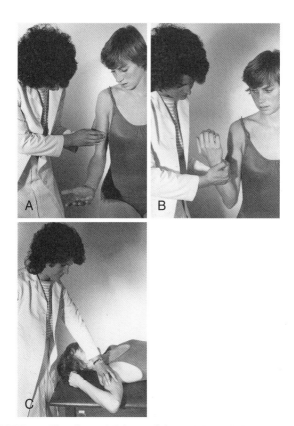

FIGURE 3-48 Elbow flexion. **A,** Palpate and observe. **B,** Resist. **C,** Gravity-minimized position.

Elbow Extension

Muscles	Innervation
Triceps	Radial nerve, C6-8
Aconeus	Radial nerve, C7,8

PROCEDURE FOR TESTING GRADES N (5) TO F (3)

1. Position: The client is prone, with the humerus abducted to 90 degrees, the elbow flexed to 90 degrees, and the forearm in neutral rotation and perpendicular to the floor. The therapist stands next to the client, just behind the arm to be tested.[7,14,20]

2. Stabilize: Provide stabilization at the humerus by placing one hand for support under it, between the client's arm and the table.[12,14]

3. Palpate: Palpate the triceps over the middle of the posterior aspect of the humerus or the triceps tendon just proximal to the olecranon process on the dorsal surface of the arm.[6,7,10,15]

4. Observe: Observe the client extending the elbow to just less than maximal range. The wrist and fingers remain relaxed.

5. Resist: Provide resistance at the distal end of the forearm into elbow flexion. Before resistance is given, be sure that the elbow is not locked. Resistance to a locked elbow can cause joint injury.

PROCEDURE FOR TESTING GRADES P (2), T (1), AND 0

1. Position: The client is supine, with the humerus abducted to 90 degrees and in external rotation, the elbow fully flexed, and the forearm supinated. The therapist is standing next to the client, just behind the arm to be tested. An alternate position is with the client seated, shoulder abducted to 90 degrees in neutral rotation, elbow flexed, and forearm in neutral position, supported by the therapist.

2. Stabilize: Provide stabilization at the humerus by holding one hand over the middle or distal end to prevent shoulder motion.

3. Palpate: Palpate the triceps as described for the previous test.

4. Observe: Observe the client extending the elbow, moving the hand away from the head.

5. Grade: The client is graded according to the standard definitions of muscle grades.

Substitutions

Finger and wrist extensors may substitute for weak elbow extensors. Observe for the presence of finger and wrist extension preceding elbow extension. When the client is upright, gravity and eccentric contraction of the biceps will effect elbow extension from the flexed position. Scapula depression, and shoulder external rotation, aided by gravity is another effective substitution pattern for elbow extension.

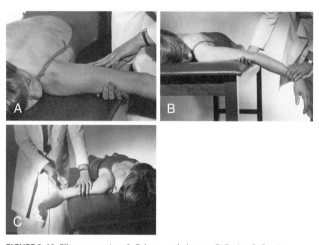

FIGURE 3-49 Elbow extension. **A,** Palpate and observe. **B,** Resist. **C,** Gravity-minimized position.

Forearm Supination

Muscles	**Innervation**
Biceps brachii	Musculocutaneous nerve, C5,6
Supinator	Radial nerve, C5-7

PROCEDURE FOR TESTING GRADES N (5) TO F (3)

1. Position: The client is seated, with the humerus adducted, the elbow flexed to 90 degrees, and the forearm pronated. The therapist stands in front of the client or next to the client on the side to be tested.
2. Stabilize: Provide stabilization at the humerus just proximal to the elbow.
3. Palpate: Palpate the client over the supinator muscle on the dorsal-lateral aspect of the forearm, below the head of the radius. The muscle can be best felt when the radial muscle group (extensor carpi radialis and brachioradialis) is pushed up out of the way. The therapist may also palpate the biceps on the middle of the anterior surface of the humerus.
4. Observe: Observe the client supinating the forearm, turning the hand palm up. Because gravity assists the movement, after the 0-degree neutral position is passed, the therapist may apply slight resistance equal to the weight of the forearm.
5. Resist: Provide resistance by grasping around the dorsal aspect of the distal forearm with the fingers and heel of the hand, turning the arm toward pronation.

PROCEDURE FOR TESTING GRADES P (2), T (1), AND 0

1. Position: The client is seated, shoulder flexed to 90 degrees and the upper arm resting on the supporting surface, elbow flexed to 90 degrees; the forearm is in full pronation in a position perpendicular to the floor. The therapist stands next to the client on the side to be tested.
2. Stabilize: Provide stabilization at the humerus just proximal to the elbow.
3. Palpate: Palpate the supinator or biceps as described for the previous test.
4. Observe: Observe the client supinating the forearm, turning the palm of the hand toward the face.
5. Grade: The client is graded according to the standard definitions of muscle grades.

Substitutions

With the elbow flexed, external rotation and horizontal adduction of the humerus will affect forearm supination. With the elbow extended, shoulder external rotation will place the forearm in supination. The brachioradialis can bring the forearm from full pronation to midposition. Wrist and thumb extensors, assisted by gravity, can initiate supination. The therapist should note any external rotation of the humerus, supination to midline only, and initiation of motion by wrist and thumb extension.

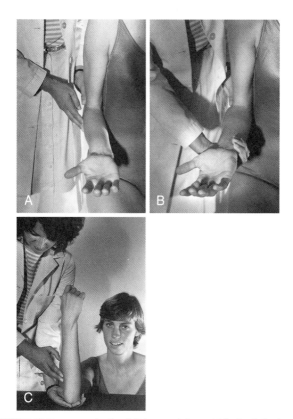

FIGURE 3-50 Forearm supination. **A,** Palpate and observe. **B,** Resist. **C,** Gravity-minimized position.

Forearm Pronation

Muscles	Innervation
Pronator teres	Median nerve, C6,7
Pronator quadratus	Median nerve, C6-8

PROCEDURE FOR TESTING GRADES N (5) TO F (3)

1. Position: The client is seated, with the humerus adducted, the elbow flexed to 90 degrees, and the forearm in full supination. The therapist stands beside the client on the side to be tested.
2. Stabilize: Provide stabilization at the humerus just proximal to the elbow to prevent shoulder abduction.
3. Palpate: Palpate the pronator teres on the upper part of the volar surface of the forearm, medial to the biceps tendon and diagonally from the medial condyle of the humerus to the lateral border of the radius.
4. Observe: Observe the client pronating the forearm, turning the hand palm down. Slight resistance may be applied after the arm has passed midposition to compensate for the assistance of gravity after that point.
5. Resist: Provide resistance by grasping over the dorsal aspect of the distal forearm, using the fingers and heel of the hand and turning toward supination.

PROCEDURE FOR TESTING GRADES P (2), T (1), AND 0

1. Position: The client is seated, shoulder flexed to 90 degrees, elbow flexed to 90 degrees, and the forearm in full supination. The upper arm is resting on the supporting surface, and the forearm is perpendicular to the floor. The therapist stands next to the client on the side to be tested.
2. Palpate: Palpate the pronator teres as described for the previous test.
3. Observe: Observe the client pronating the forearm, turning the palm of the hand away from the face.
4. Grade: The client is graded according to the standard definitions of muscle grades.

Substitutions

With the elbow flexed, internal rotation and abduction of the humerus will produce apparent forearm pronation. With the elbow extended, internal rotation can place the forearm in a pronated position. Brachioradialis can bring the fully supinated forearm to midposition. Wrist flexion, aided by gravity, can effect pronation.

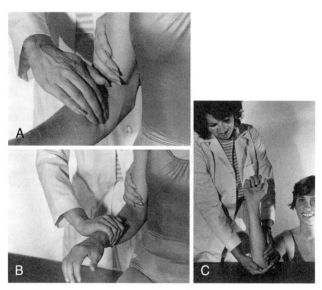

FIGURE 3-51 Forearm pronation. **A,** Palpate and observe. **B,** Resist. **C,** Gravity-minimized position.

Wrist Extension with Radial Deviation

Muscles   **Innervation**
Extensor carpi radialis longus (ECRL)   Radial nerve, C5-7
Extensor carpi radialis brevis (ECRB)   Radial nerve, C6-8
Extensor carpi ulnaris (ECU)

PROCEDURE FOR TESTING GRADES N (5) TO F (3)

1. Position: The client is seated or supine, with the forearm resting on the supporting surface in pronation, the wrist at neutral, and the fingers and thumb relaxed. The therapist sits opposite to or next to the client on the side to be tested.
2. Stabilize: Provide stabilization over the volar or dorsal aspect of the distal forearm.
3. Palpate: Palpate the ECRL and ECRB tendons on the dorsal aspect of the wrist at the bases of the second and third metacarpals, respectively. The tendon of the ECU may be palpated at the base of the fifth metacarpal, just distal to the head of the ulna.
4. Observe: Observe the client extending and radially deviating the wrist, lifting the hand from the supporting surface and simultaneously moving it medially (to the radial side). The movement should be performed without finger extension, which could substitute for the wrist motion.
5. Resist: Provide resistance over the dorsum of the second and third metacarpals, toward flexion and ulnar deviation.

PROCEDURE FOR TESTING GRADES P (2), T (1), AND 0

1. Position: The client is placed in the same manner as described for the previous test, except that the forearm is resting in midposition on its ulnar border.
2. Stabilize: Provide stabilization at the ulnar border of the forearm, supported slightly above the table surface.
3. Palpate: Palpate radial wrist extensors, as described for the previous test.
4. Observe: Observe client extending the wrist, moving the hand away from the body.
5. Grade: The client is graded according to the standard definitions of muscle grades.

Substitutions

Wrist extensors can substitute for one another. In the absence of the extensor carpi radialis muscles, the extensor carpi ulnaris will extend the wrist, but in an ulnar direction. The combined extension and radial deviation will not be possible. The extensor digitorum communis muscle and the extensor pollicis longus can initiate wrist extension, but finger or thumb extension will precede wrist extension.

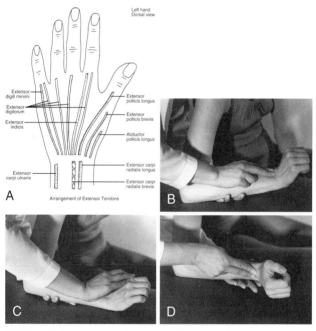

FIGURE 3-52 A, Arrangement of extensor tendons at wrist. **B,** Wrist extension with radial deviation. Palpate and observe. **C,** Resist. **D,** Gravity-minimized position.

Wrist Extension with Ulnar Deviation

Muscles	Innervation
Extensor carpi ulnaris (ECU)	Radial nerve, C6-8
Extensor carpi radialis brevis (ECRB)	
Extensor carpi radialis longus (ECRL)	Radial nerve, C5-7

PROCEDURE FOR TESTING GRADES N (5) TO F (3)

1. Position: The client is seated, forearm pronated, wrist neutral, fingers and thumb relaxed, supported on a table. The therapist sits opposite or next to the client on the side to be tested.
2. Stabilize: Provide stabilization under the distal forearm.
3. Palpate: Palpate the ECU tendon at the base of the fifth metacarpal, just distal to the ulnar styloid, and the ECRL and ECRB tendons at the bases of the second and third metacarpals.
4. Observe: Observe the client extending the wrist and simultaneously moving it laterally (to the ulnar side). The therapist should observe that the movement is not preceded by thumb or finger extension.
5. Resist: Provide resistance over the dorsal-lateral aspect of the fourth and fifth metacarpals toward flexion and radial deviation.

PROCEDURE FOR TESTING GRADES P (2), T (1), AND 0

1. Position: The client is placed in the same manner as that described for the previous test, except that the forearm is in 45 degrees of pronation and supported on a table. The wrist is flexed and radially deviated, and the thumb and fingers are flexed.
2. Stabilize: Provide stabilization under the distal forearm, supporting it slightly above the supporting surface.
3. Palpate: Palpate the extensor tendons, as described earlier.
4. Observe: Observe client extending the wrist and moving it ulnarly at the same time.
5. Grade: The client is graded according to the standard definitions of muscle grades.

Substitutions

In the absence of the ECU muscle, the ECRL and ECRB muscles can extend the wrist but will do so in a radial direction. The ulnar deviation component of the test motion will not be possible. Long finger and thumb extensors can initiate wrist extension, but the movement will be preceded by finger or thumb extension.

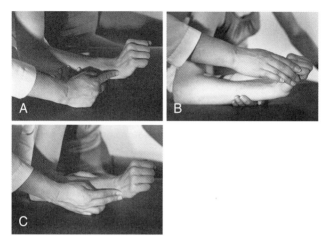

FIGURE 3-53 Wrist extension with ulnar deviation. **A,** Palpate and observe. **B,** Resist. **C,** Gravity-minimized position.

Wrist Flexion with Radial Deviation

Muscles	Innervation
Flexor carpi radialis (FCR)	Median nerve, C6-8
Flexor carpi ulnaris (FCU)	Ulnar nerve, C7-T1
Palmaris longus	Median nerve, C7-T1

PROCEDURE FOR TESTING GRADES N (5) TO F (3)

1. Position: The client is seated or supine, with the forearm resting in almost full supination on the supporting surface, fingers and thumb relaxed. The therapist is seated next to the client on the side to be tested.
2. Stabilize: Provide stabilization over the volar aspect of the midforearm.
3. Palpate: The FCR tendon can be palpated over the wrist at the base of the second metacarpal bone. The palmaris longus tendon is at the center of the wrist at the base of the third metacarpal, and the FCU tendon can be palpated at the ulnar side of the volar aspect of the wrist, at the base of the fifth metacarpal.

4. Observe: Observe the client simultaneously flexing and radially deviating the hand. The therapist should observe that the fingers remain relaxed during the movement.
5. Resist: Provide resistance in the palm at the radial side of the hand, over the second and third metacarpals, toward extension and ulnar deviation.

PROCEDURE FOR TESTING GRADES P (2), T (1), AND 0

1. Position: The client is seated with the forearm in midposition and the ulnar border of the hand resting on the supporting surface. The therapist sits next to the client on the side to be tested.
2. Stabilize: Provide stabilization under the ulnar border of the forearm, supporting the wrist slightly above the supporting surface.
3. Palpate: Palpate the wrist flexor tendons as described for the previous test.
4. Observe: Observe the client flexing and radially deviating the wrist. Movement should not be initiated with finger flexion.
5. Grade: The client is graded according to the standard definitions of muscle grades.

Substitutions

Wrist flexors can substitute for one another. If the flexor carpi radialis is weak or nonfunctioning in this test, the flexor carpi ulnaris will produce wrist flexion, but in an ulnar direction, and the radial deviation will not be possible. The finger flexors can assist wrist flexion, but finger flexion will occur before the wrist is flexed. The abductor pollicis longus, with the assistance of gravity, can initiate wrist flexion.

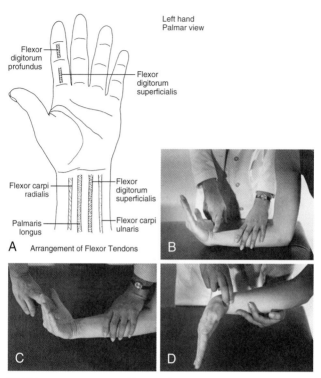

FIGURE 3-54 A, Arrangement of flexor tendons at wrist. **B,** Wrist flexion with radial deviation. Palpate and observe. **C,** Resist. **D,** Gravity-minimized position.

Wrist Flexion with Ulnar Deviation

Muscles
Flexor carpi ulnaris (FCU)
Palmaris longus
Flexor carpi radialis (FCR)

Innervation
Ulnar nerve, C7-T1
Median nerve, C7-T1
Median nerve, C6-8

PROCEDURE FOR TESTING GRADES N (5) TO F (3)

1. Position: The client is seated or supine, with the forearm resting in almost full supination on the supporting surface, fingers and

thumb relaxed. The therapist is seated opposite or next to the client on the side to be tested.

2. Stabilize: Provide stabilization over the volar aspect of the middle of the forearm.

3. Palpate: Palpate the flexor tendons on the volar aspect of the wrist, the FCU at the base of the fifth metacarpal, the FCR at the base of the second metacarpal, and the palmaris longus at the base of the third metacarpal.

4. Observe: Observe the client simultaneously flexing the wrist and deviating it ulnarly.

5. Resist: Provide resistance in the palm of the hand over the hypothenar eminence toward extension and radial deviation.

PROCEDURE FOR TESTING GRADES P (2), T (1), AND 0

1. Position: The client is seated with the forearm in neutral rotation and resting in 45 degrees of supination on the ulnar border of the arm and hand. The therapist sits opposite or next to the client on the side being tested.

2. Stabilize: The client's arm can be supported slightly above the supporting surface and stabilized at the dorsal-medial aspect of the forearm to prevent elbow and forearm motion.

3. Palpate: Palpate the wrist flexor tendons as described for the previous test.

4. Observe: Observe the client simultaneously flexing and deviating the wrist toward ulnar side.

5. Grade: The client is graded according to the standard definitions of muscle grades.

Substitutions

Wrist flexors can substitute for one another. If the FCU is weak or absent, the FCR can produce wrist flexion in a radial direction and the ulnar deviation will not be possible. The finger flexors can also assist wrist flexion, but the motion will be preceded by flexion of the fingers.

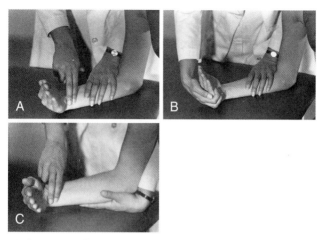

FIGURE 3-55 Wrist flexion with ulnar deviation. **A,** Palpate and observe. **B,** Resist. **C,** Gravity-minimized position.

Metacarpophalangeal Flexion with Interphalangeal Extension

Muscles	Innervation
Lumbricals 1 and 2	Median nerve, C8,T1
Lumbricals 3 and 4	Ulnar nerve, C8,T1
Dorsal interossei	
Palmar interossei	

PROCEDURE FOR TESTING GRADES N (5) TO F (3)

1. Position: The client is seated, with forearm in supination, wrist at neutral, resting on the supporting surface. The metacarpophalangeal (MP) joints are extended and the interphalangeal (IP) joints are flexed. The therapist sits next to the client on the side being tested.
2. Stabilize: Provide stabilization over the metacarpals, proximal to the MP joints in the palm of the hand to prevent wrist motion.
3. Palpate: Palpate the first dorsal interosseous muscle just medial to the distal aspect of the second metacarpal on the dorsum of the hand. The remainder of these muscles are not easily palpable because of their size and deep location in the hand.

4. Observe: Observe the client flexing the MP joints and extending the IP joints simultaneously.
5. Resist: Provide resistance to each finger separately by grasping the distal phalanx and pushing downward on the finger into the supporting surface toward MP extension and IP flexion, or apply pressure first against the dorsal surface of the middle and distal phalanges toward flexion, followed by application of pressure to the volar surface of the proximal phalanges toward extension.

PROCEDURE FOR TESTING GRADES P (2), T (1), AND 0

1. Position: The client is seated or supine, with the forearm and wrist in midposition and resting on the ulnar border on the supporting surface. The MP joints are extended and the IP joints are flexed. The therapist sits next to the client on the side being tested.
2. Stabilize: Provide stabilization at the wrist and palm of the hand.
3. Palpate: Palpate the client as described for the previous test.
4. Observe: Observe the client flexing the MP joints and extending the IP joints simultaneously.
5. Grade: The client is graded according to the standard definitions of muscle grades.

Substitutions
The flexor digitorum profundus and superficialis may substitute for weak or absent lumbricals. In this case, MP flexion will be preceded by flexion of the distal and proximal IP joints.

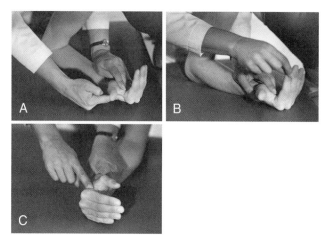

FIGURE 3-56 Metacarpophalangeal flexion with interphalangeal extension. **A,** Palpate and observe. **B,** Resist. **C,** Gravity-minimized position.

Metacarpophalangeal Extension

Muscles
Extensor digitorum communis (EDC)
Extensor indicis
Extensor digiti minimi (EDM)

Innervation
Radial nerve, C7,8

PROCEDURE FOR TESTING GRADES N (5) TO F (3)

1. Position: The client is seated, with the forearm pronated and the wrist in the neutral position, and the MP and IP joints relaxed and in partial flexion. The therapist sits opposite or next to the client on the side to be tested.
2. Stabilize: Provide stabilization at the wrist and metacarpals slightly above the supporting surface.
3. Palpate: Palpate the EDC tendons where they course over the dorsum of the hand. In some individuals, the EDM tendon can be palpated or visualized just lateral to the EDC tendon to the fifth finger. The extensor indicis tendon can be palpated or visualized just medial to the EDC tendon to the first finger.
4. Observe: Observe the client extending the MP joints but maintaining the IP joints in some flexion.

5. Resist: Provide resistance to each finger individually on the dorsum of the proximal phalanx toward MP flexion.

PROCEDURE FOR TESTING GRADES P (2), T (1), AND 0

1. Position: The patient should be placed in a position similar to that described for the previous test, except that the client's forearm is in midposition and the hand and forearm are supported on the ulnar border.
2. Stabilize: Provide stabilization in the same manner as described for the previous test.
3. Palpate: Palpate the patient in the same manner as described for the previous test.
4. Observe: Observe the client extending the MP joints while keeping the IP joints somewhat flexed.
5. Grade: The patient is graded according to the standard definitions of muscle grades.

Substitutions

With the wrist stabilized, no substitutions are possible. When the wrist is not stabilized, wrist flexion with tendon action can produce MP extension.

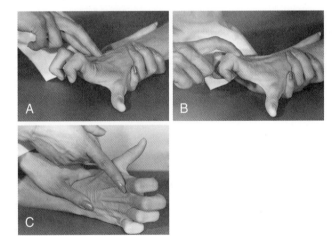

FIGURE 3-57 Metacarpophalangeal extension. **A,** Palpate and observe. **B,** Resist. **C,** Gravity-minimized position.

Proximal Interphalangeal Flexion, Second Through Fifth Fingers

Muscles
Flexor digitorum superficialis

Innervation
Median nerve, C7,8,T1 (FDS)

PROCEDURE FOR TESTING GRADES N (5) TO F (3)

1. Position: The client is seated, with the forearm supinated, wrist at neutral, fingers extended, and hand and forearm resting on the dorsal surface. The therapist sits opposite or next to the client on the side being tested.
2. Stabilize: Provide stabilization at the MP joint and proximal phalanx of the finger being tested. If it is difficult for the client to isolate PIP flexion, hold all the fingers not being tested in MP hyperextension and PIP extension. This maneuver inactivates the flexor digitorum profundus so that the client cannot flex the distal joint. Most individuals cannot perform isolated action of the PIP joint of the fifth finger, even with this assistance.
3. Palpate: Palpate the FDS tendon on the volar surface of the proximal phalanx. A stabilizing finger may be used to palpate in this case. The tendon supplying the fourth finger may be palpated over the volar aspect of the wrist between the flexor carpi ulnaris and the palmaris longus tendons, if desired.
4. Observe: Observe the client flexing the PIP joint while maintaining DIP extension.
5. Resist: Provide resistance with one finger at the volar aspect of the middle phalanx toward extension. If the therapist uses the index finger to apply resistance, the middle finger may be used to move the DIP joint to and fro to verify that the flexor digitorum profundus (FDP) is not substituting.

PROCEDURE FOR TESTING GRADES P (2), T (1), AND 0

1. Position: The client is seated, with the forearm in midposition and the wrist at neutral, resting on the ulnar border. The therapist sits opposite or next to the client on the side to be tested.
2. Stabilize: Provide stabilization at the MP joint and proximal phalanx of the finger. If stabilization during the motion is difficult in this position, the forearm may be returned to full supination because the effect of gravity on the fingers is not significant.

3. Palpate and observe: The therapist palpates and observes the client in the same manner as described for the previous test, except that the movement is performed in the gravity-minimized position.
4. Grade: The client is graded according to the standard definitions of muscle grades. If the test for grades poor and below is done with the forearm in full supination, partial ROM against gravity may be graded poor.

Substitutions

The FDP may substitute for the FDS. DIP flexion will precede PIP flexion. Tendon action of the long finger flexors accompanies wrist extension and can produce an apparent flexion of the fingers through partial ROM.

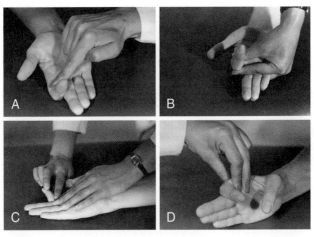

FIGURE 3-58 Proximal interphalangeal flexion. **A,** Palpate and observe. **B,** Position to assist with isolation of proximal interphalangeal joint flexion. **C,** Resist. Therapist checks for substitution by flexor digitorum profundus. **D,** Gravity-minimized position.

Distal Interphalangeal Flexion, Second Through Fifth Fingers

Muscles
Flexor digitorum profundus

Innervation
Median and ulnar nerves, (FDP)
C8, T1

PROCEDURE FOR TESTING GRADES N (5) TO F (3)

1. Position: The client is seated, with the forearm supinated, the wrist at neutral, and the fingers extended. The therapist sits opposite or next to the client on the side being tested.
2. Stabilize: Provide stabilization at the wrist at neutral and the PIP joint and middle phalanx of the finger being tested.
3. Palpate: Use the finger stabilizing the middle phalanx to palpate the FDP tendon simultaneously over the volar surface of the middle phalanx.
4. Observe: Observe the client flexing the DIP joint.
5. Resist: Provide resistance with one finger at the volar aspect of the distal phalanx toward extension.

PROCEDURE FOR TESTING GRADES P (2), T (1), AND 0

1. Position: The client is seated, with the forearm in midposition and with the wrist at neutral, resting on the ulnar border. The client may be positioned with the forearm supinated, if necessary.
2. Stabilize: The client is stabilized in the same manner as described for the previous test.
3. Palpate: The client is palpated in the same manner as described for the previous test.
4. Observe: Observe the client flexing the DIP joint.
5. Grade: The client is graded according to the standard definitions of muscle grades, except that if the test for grades poor and below was done with the forearm in full supination, movement through partial ROM may be graded poor.

Substitutions

There are none possible during the testing procedure if the wrist is well stabilized because the FDP is the only muscle that can act to flex the DIP joint when it is isolated. During normal hand function, however, wrist extension with tendon action of the finger flexors can produce partial flexion of the DIP joints.

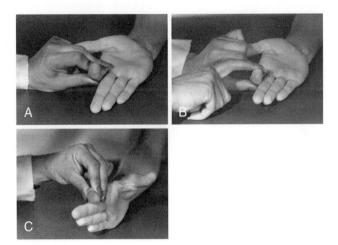

FIGURE 3-59 Distal interphalangeal flexion. **A,** Palpate and observe. **B,** Resist. **C,** Gravity-minimized position.

Finger Abduction

Muscles
Dorsal interossei
Abductor digiti minimi

Innervation
Ulnar nerve, C8,T1

PROCEDURE FOR TESTING GRADES N (5) TO F (3)

1. Position: The client is seated or supine, with the forearm pronated, wrist at neutral, and fingers extended and adducted. The therapist is seated opposite or next to the client on the side to be tested.
2. Stabilize: Provide stabilization at the wrist and metacarpals slightly above the supporting surface.
3. Palpate: Palpate the first dorsal interosseous muscle on the radial side of the second metacarpal or of the abductor digiti minimi on the ulnar border of the fifth metacarpal. The remaining interossei are not palpable.
4. Observe: Observe the client spreading the fingers—abduction of the little finger, the ring finger toward the little finger, the middle

finger toward the ring finger, and the index finger toward the thumb.

5. Resist: Provide the first dorsal interosseous by applying pressure on the radial side of the proximal phalanx of the second finger in an ulnar direction, the second dorsal interosseous on the radial side of the proximal phalanx of the middle finger in an ulnar direction, the third dorsal interosseous on the ulnar side of the proximal phalanx of the middle finger in a radial direction, the fourth dorsal interosseous on the ulnar side of the proximal phalanx of the ring finger in a radial direction, and the abductor digiti minimi on the ulnar side of the proximal phalanx of the little finger in a radial direction. An alternative mode of resistance is to flick each finger toward adduction. If the finger rebounds, the grade is N (5).

PROCEDURE FOR TESTING GRADES P (2), T (1), AND 0

The tests for these muscle grades are the same as described for the previous test.

1. Grade: Because the test motions were not performed against gravity, the therapist must exercise professional judgment when grading. For example, partial ROM in the gravity-minimized position may be graded poor and full ROM graded fair.

Substitutions

The EDC can assist weak or absent dorsal interossei, but abduction will be accompanied by MP extension.

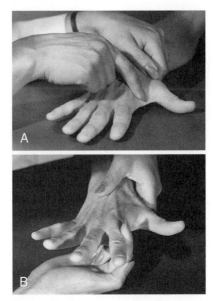

FIGURE 3-60 Finger abduction. **A,** Palpate and observe. **B,** Resist.

Finger Adduction

Muscles
Palmar interossei, 1, 2, 3

Innervation
Ulnar nerve, C8,T1

PROCEDURE FOR TESTING GRADES N (5) TO F (3)

1. Position: The client is seated, with the forearm pronated, wrist in neutral, and fingers extended and abducted.
2. Stabilize: Provide stabilization at the wrist and metacarpals slightly above the supporting surface.
3. Palpate: The condition is not palpable. The muscle cannot be palpated.
4. Observe: Observe the client adducting the first, fourth, and fifth fingers toward the middle finger.
5. Resist: Provide resistance at the index finger at the proximal phalanx by pulling it in a radial direction, the ring finger at the

proximal phalanx in an ulnar direction, and the little finger similarly. These muscles are very small and resistance must be modified to accommodate their comparatively limited power. Fingers can also be grasped at the distal phalanx and flicked in the direction of abduction. If the finger snaps back to the adducted position, the grade is N (5).

PROCEDURE FOR TESTING GRADES P (2), T (1), AND 0

The test for these muscle grades is the same as described for the previous test. The therapist's judgment must be used in determining the degree of weakness. Achievement of full ROM may be graded fair and partial ROM graded poor.

Substitutions
The FDP and FDS can substitute for weak palmar interossei, but IP flexion will occur with finger adduction.

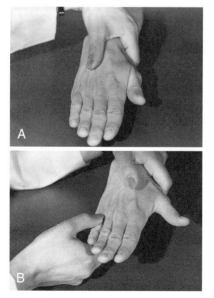

FIGURE 3-61 Finger adduction. **A,** Therapist observes movement of fingers into adduction. Palpation of these muscles is not possible. **B,** Resist.

Thumb Metacarpophalangeal Extension

Muscles
Extensor pollicis brevis (EPB)

Innervation
Radial nerve, C6-8

PROCEDURE FOR TESTING GRADES N (5) TO F (3)

1. Position: The client is seated or supine, forearm in midposition, wrist at neutral, and hand and forearm resting on the ulnar border. The thumb is flexed into the palm at the MP joint, and the IP joint is extended but relaxed. The therapist sits opposite or next to the client on the side to be tested.
2. Stabilize: Provide stabilization at the wrist and the thumb metacarpal.
3. Palpate: Palpate the EPB tendon on the dorsoradial aspect of the base of the first metacarpal. It lies just medial to the abductor pollicis longus tendon on the radial side of the anatomic snuffbox, which is the hollow space created between the EPL and EPB tendons when the thumb is fully extended and radially abducted.
4. Observe: Observe the client extending the MP joint. The IP joint remains relaxed. It is difficult for many individuals to isolate this motion.
5. Resist: Provide resistance on the dorsal surface of the proximal phalanx toward MP flexion.

PROCEDURE FOR TESTING GRADES (P), (T), AND (0)

1. Position and stabilize: Positioning and stabilizing are the same as described for the previous test, except that the forearm is fully pronated and resting on the volar surface. The therapist may stabilize the first metacarpal, holding the hand slightly above the supporting surface. The test may also be performed in the same manner as for grades normal to fair, with modified grading.
2. Palpate and observe: The client is palpated and observed in the same way as described for the previous test. MP extension is performed in a plane parallel to the supporting surface.
3. Grade: The client is graded according to the standard definitions of muscle grades. If midposition of the forearm was used, partial ROM is graded poor and full ROM is graded fair.

Substitutions
The extensor pollicis longus may substitute for extensor pollicis brevis. IP extension will precede MP extension.

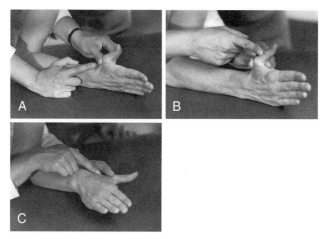

FIGURE 3-62 Thumb metacarpophalangeal extension. **A,** Palpate and observe. **B,** Resist. **C,** Gravity-minimized position.

Thumb IP Extension

Muscles
Extensor pollicis longus (EPL)

Innervation
Radial nerve, C6-8

PROCEDURE FOR TESTING GRADES N (5) TO F (3)

1. Position: The client is seated or supine, forearm in midposition, wrist at neutral, and hand and forearm resting on the ulnar border. The thumb is adducted, the MP joint is extended or slightly flexed, and the IP is flexed. The therapist sits opposite or next to the client on the side being tested.
2. Stabilize: Provide stabilization at the wrist in neutral position, the first metacarpal, and the proximal phalanx of the thumb.
3. Palpate: Palpate the EPL tendon on the dorsal surface of the hand medial to the EPB tendon, between the head of the first metacarpal and the base of the second on the ulnar side of the anatomic snuffbox.
4. Observe: C extend the IP joint.
5. Resist: Provide resistance on the dorsal surface of the distal phalanx, down toward IP flexion.

PROCEDURE FOR TESTING GRADES P (2), T (1), AND 0

1. Position and stabilize: Positioning and stabilizing are the same as described for the previous test, except that the forearm is fully pronated. The therapist may stabilize so that the client's hand is held slightly above the supporting surface. The test may also be performed in the same position as for grades normal to fair with modification in grading.
2. Palpate and observe: The patient is palpated and observed in the same manner as described for the previous test. IP extension is performed in the plane of the palm, parallel to the supporting surface.
3. Grade: The client is graded according to the standard definitions of muscle grades. If the test was performed with the forearm in midposition, partial ROM is graded P (2).

Substitutions

A quick contraction of the flexor pollicis longus followed by rapid release will cause the IP joint to rebound into extension. IP flexion will precede IP extension. The abductor pollicis brevis, flexor pollicis brevis, oblique fibers of the adductor pollicis, and first palmar interosseous can extend the IP joint because of their insertions into the extensor expansion of the thumb.

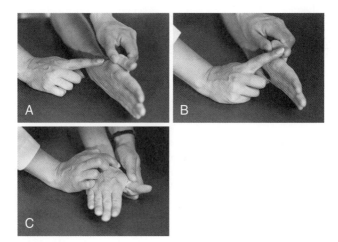

FIGURE 3-63 Thumb interphalangeal extension. **A,** Palpate and observe. **B,** Resist. **C,** Gravity-minimized position.

Thumb Metacarpophalangeal Flexion

Muscles
Flexor pollicis brevis (FPB)

Innervation
Median and ulnar nerves, C8, T1

PROCEDURE FOR TESTING GRADES N (5) TO F (3)

1. Position: The client is seated or supine, the forearm supinated, the wrist in the neutral position, and the thumb in extension and adduction. The therapist is seated next to or opposite the client.
2. Stabilize: Provide stabilization at the first metacarpal and the wrist.
3. Palpate: Palpate the client over the middle of the palmar surface of the thenar eminence just medial to the abductor pollicis brevis muscle. The hand that is used to stabilize may also be used for palpation.
4. Observe: Observe the client flexing the MP joint while maintaining extension of the IP joint. It may not be possible for some individuals to isolate flexion to the MP joint. In this case, both MP and IP flexion may be tested together as a gross test for thumb flexion strength and graded according to the therapist's judgment.
5. Resist: Provide resistance on the palmar surface of the first phalanx toward MP extension.

PROCEDURE FOR TESTING GRADES P (2), T (1), AND (0)

Positioning, stabilizing, and palpating are the same as described for the previous test.

1. Observe: Observe the client flexing the MP joint so that the thumb moves over the palm of the hand.
2. Grade: Full ROM is graded fair; partial ROM is graded poor.

Substitutions
FPL can substitute for FPB. In this case, isolated MP flexion will not be possible and MP flexion will be preceded by IP flexion.

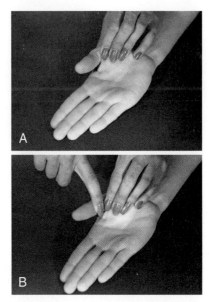

FIGURE 3-64 Thumb metacarpophalangeal flexion. **A,** Palpate and observe. **B,** Resist.

Thumb Interphalangeal Flexion

Muscles
Flexor pollicis longus (FPL)

Innervation
Median nerve, C7-T1

PROCEDURE FOR TESTING GRADES N (5) TO F (3)

1. Position: The client is seated, with the forearm fully supinated, wrist in neutral position, and thumb extended and adducted. The therapist is seated next to or opposite the client.
2. Stabilize: Provide stabilization at the wrist, thumb metacarpal, and proximal phalanx of the thumb in extension.
3. Palpate: Palpate the FPL tendon on the palmar surface of the proximal phalanx. In this case, the palpating finger may be the same one used for stabilizing the proximal phalanx.
4. Observe: Observe the client flexing the IP joint in the plane of the palm.

5. Resist: Provide resistance on the palmar surface of the distal phalanx, toward IP extension.

PROCEDURE FOR TESTING GRADES P (2), T (1), AND 0

The test for these muscle grades is the same as that described for the previous test. The OT's judgment must be used in determining the degree of weakness. Achievement of full ROM may be graded fair and partial ROM graded poor.

Substitutions

A quick contraction and release of the EPL may cause an apparent flexion of the IP joint. The therapist should observe for IP extension preceding IP flexion.

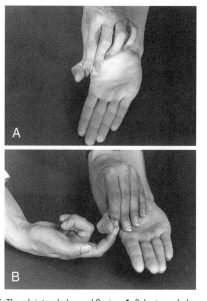

FIGURE 3-65 Thumb interphalangeal flexion. **A,** Palpate and observe. **B,** Resist.

Thumb Palmar Abduction

Muscles
Abductor pollicis brevis (APB)

Innervation
Median nerve, C8,T1

PROCEDURE FOR TESTING GRADES FAIR (F) TO NORMAL (N)

1. Position: The client is seated or supine, forearm in supination, wrist at neutral, thumb relaxed in adduction against the volar aspect of the index finger. The OT sits opposite or next to the client on the side to be tested.
2. Stabilize: Provide stabilization at the metacarpals and wrist.
3. Palpate: Palpate the APB muscle on the lateral aspect of the thenar eminence, lateral to the flexor pollicis brevis muscle.
4. Observe: Observe the client raising the thumb away from the palm in a plane perpendicular to the palm.
5. Resist: Provide resistance at the lateral aspect of the proximal phalanx, downward toward adduction.

PROCEDURE FOR TESTING GRADES P (2), T (1), AND 0

1. Position: The client is positioned in the same manner as described for the previous test, except that the forearm and hand are supported on the ulnar border.
2. Stabilize: Provide stabilization at the wrist and metacarpals.
3. Palpate: Palpate the APB muscle on the lateral aspect of the thenar eminence.
4. Observe: Observe the client moving the thumb away from the palm in a plane at right angles to the palm of the hand and parallel to the supporting surface.
5. Grade: The client is graded according to the standard definitions of muscle grades.

Substitutions

The APL can substitute for the APB. Abduction will take place more in the plane of the palm, however, rather than perpendicular to it.

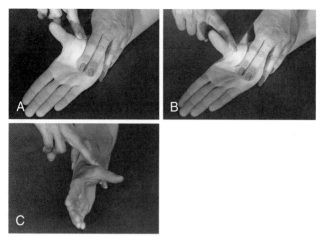

FIGURE 3-66 Thumb palmar abduction. **A,** Palpate and observe. **B,** Resist. **C,** Gravity-minimized position.

Thumb Radial Abduction

Muscles
Abductor pollicis longus (APL)

Innervation
Radial nerve, C6-8

PROCEDURE FOR TESTING GRADES N (5) TO F (3)

1. Position: The client is seated or supine, forearm in neutral rotation, wrist at neutral, thumb adducted and slightly flexed across the palm. The hand and forearm are resting on the ulnar border. The therapist sits opposite or next to the client on the side being tested.
2. Stabilize: Provide stabilization at the wrist and metacarpals of the fingers.
3. Palpate: Palpate the APL tendon on the lateral aspect of the base of the first metacarpal. It is the tendon immediately lateral (radial) to the EPB tendon.
4. Observe: Observe the client moving the thumb out of the palm of the hand, abducting away from the index finger at an angle of approximately 45 degrees.
5. Resist: Provide resistance at the lateral aspect of the thumb metacarpal toward adduction.

PROCEDURE FOR TESTING GRADES P (2), T (1), AND 0

1. Position: The client is positioned in the same manner as described for the previous test, except that the forearm is in supination.
2. Stabilize: Provide stabilization at the wrist and palm of the hand.
3. Palpate: The client is palpated in the same manner as described for the previous test.
4. Observe: Observe the client moving the thumb out away from the palm of the hand in the plane of the palm.
5. Grade: The client is graded according to the standard definitions of muscle grades.

Substitutions

The APB can substitute for the APL. Abduction will not take place in the plane of the palm but rather in a more ulnar direction. EPB can substitute for APL. The movement will be more toward the dorsal surface of the forearm.[12]

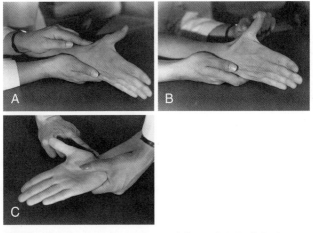

FIGURE 3-67 Radial abduction. **A,** Palpate and observe. **B,** Resist. **C,** Gravity-minimized position.

Thumb Adduction

Muscles   **Innervation**
Adductor pollicis (AP)   Ulnar nerve, C8,T1

PROCEDURE FOR TESTING GRADES N (5) TO F (3)

1. Position: The client is seated or supine, forearm pronated, wrist at neutral, thumb relaxed and in palmar abduction. The therapist is sitting opposite or next to the client on the side to be tested.
2. Stabilize: Provide stabilization at the wrist and metacarpals by grasping the hand around the ulnar side and supporting it slightly above the resting surface.
3. Palpate: Palpate the AP on the palmar side of the thumb web space.
4. Observe: Observe the client adducting the thumb to touch the palm. (The palm is turned up in Figure 3-67, *C* to show the palpation point.)
5. Resist: Provide resistance by grasping the proximal phalanx of the thumb near the metacarpal head and pulling downward, toward abduction.

PROCEDURE FOR TESTING GRADES P (2), T (1), AND 0

1. Position: The client is positioned in the same manner as described for the previous test, except that the forearm is in midposition and the forearm and hand are resting on the ulnar border.
2. Stabilize: Provide stabilization over the wrist and palm of the hand.
3. Palpate: Palpate the client in the same manner as described for the previous test.
4. Observe: Observe the client adducting the thumb to touch the radial side of the palm of the hand or the second metacarpal.
5. Grade: The client is graded according to the standard definitions of muscle grades.

Substitutions

The FPL or EPL may assist a weak or absent AP. If one substitutes, adduction will be accompanied by thumb flexion or extension preceding adduction.

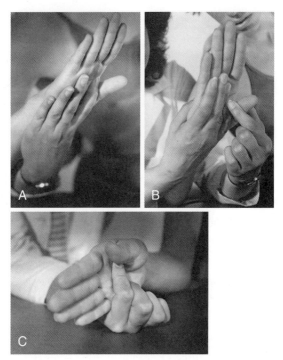

FIGURE 3-68 Thumb adduction. **A,** Palpate and observe. **B,** Resist. **C,** Gravity-minimized position.

Opposition of the Thumb to the Fifth Finger

Muscles	Innervation
Opponens pollicis	Median nerve, C8, T1
Opponens digiti minimi	Ulnar nerve, C8, T1

PROCEDURE FOR TESTING GRADES N (5) TO F (3)

1. Position: The client is seated or supine, with the forearm supinated, wrist at neutral, thumb in palmar abduction, and fifth finger extended. The therapist sits opposite or next to the client on the side to be tested.
2. Stabilize: Provide stabilization at the forearm and wrist.

3. Palpate: Palpate the opponens pollicis along the radial side of the shaft of the first metacarpal, lateral to the APB, and the opponens digiti minimi on the shaft of the fifth metacarpal.

4. Observe: Observe the client opposing the thumb to touch the thumb pad to the pad of the fifth finger, which flexes and rotates toward the thumb.

5. Resist: Provide resistance at the distal ends of the first and fifth metacarpals toward derotation of these bones and flattening of the palm of the hand.

PROCEDURE FOR TESTING GRADES P (2), T (1), AND 0

The procedure described for the previous test may be used for these grades, if grading is modified to compensate for the movement of the parts against gravity. For example, movement through full ROM would be graded fair and through partial ROM would be graded poor.

Substitutions

The APB will assist with opposition by flexing and medially rotating the carpometacarpal (CMC) joint, but the IP joint will extend. The FPB will flex and medially rotate the CMC joint, but the thumb will not move away from the palm of the hand. The FPL will flex and slightly rotate the CMC joint, but the thumb will not move away from the palm and the IP joint will flex strongly. The DIP joints of the thumb and little finger may flex to meet, giving the appearance of full opposition.

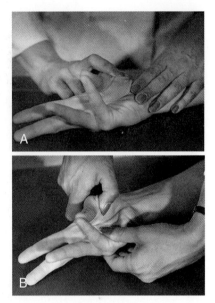

FIGURE 3-69 Thumb opposition. **A,** Palpate and observe. **B,** Resist.

Evaluation of Sensation and Intervention for Sensory Dysfunction

All clients with sensory dysfunction, regardless of the cause, should be evaluated to determine the occupational impact of the loss. The specific sensory tests and interventions may vary, according to the diagnosis and prognosis for recovery. The battery of tests selected depends on whether the diagnosis is central nervous system (CNS) or peripheral nervous system (PNS) in origin. A person with CNS injury is more likely to have deficits in proprioception and stereognosis. A person with PNS injury is more likely to have deficits in touch pressure awareness and two-point discrimination.

Somatosensory receptors are specialized to respond to stimulation of a specific nature. These receptors are categorized as mechanoreceptors, chemoreceptors, and thermoreceptors. Mechanoreceptors respond to touch, pressure, stretch, and vibration and are stimulated by mechanical deformation. Chemoreceptors respond to cell injury or damage and are stimulated by substances that the injured cells release. Thermoreceptors respond to the stimulation of heating or cooling. Each of these three types of receptors has a subset called nociceptors, which sense pain when stimulated.

Disturbances of somatosensation may present as paresthesia, hyperalgesia, dysesthesia, or allodynia. Paresthesia is a tingling, electrical, or prickling sensation. Tapping the volar aspect of the wrist may elicit paresthesias in the distribution of the median nerve in a person who has carpal tunnel syndrome. When this tapping elicits paresthesia, it is referred to as a Tinel sign. Hyperalgesia is increased pain and may occur during nerve regeneration. Hypersensitivity is increased sensory pain. Mary experienced hypersensitivity at her incision site following her surgery. Desensitization helps normalize the phenomenon of hypersensitivity. Dysesthesia is an unpleasant sensation that may be spontaneous or stimulated. Allodynia is pain in response to a stimulus that is not normally painful. An example of allodynia would be seen when a person with complex regional pain syndrome (also referred to as RSD) experiences pain with the mere movement of air wafting over the involved arm.

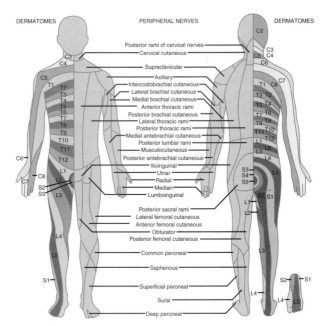

FIGURE 3-70 Cutaneous sensory distribution and dermatomes. (From Lundy-Ekman L: *Neuroscience: Fundamentals for rehabilitation,* 3rd ed. St. Louis, 2007, WB Saunders, p 109.)

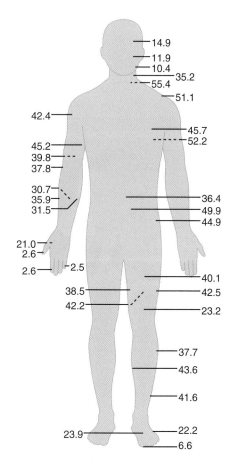

FIGURE 3-71 Normal two-point discrimination values over different locations of the body. (From Lundy-Ekman L: *Neuroscience: Fundamentals for rehabilitation,* 3rd ed. St. Louis, 2007, WB Saunders, p 134.)

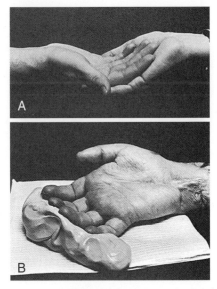

FIGURE 3-72 Ways to support the hand during sensory testing. **A,** In the examiner's hand. **B,** In putty. (From Callahan AD: Sensibility assessment for nerve lesions-in-continuity and nerve lacerations. In Skirven TM, Osterman AL, Fedorczyk J, et al (eds): *Rehabilitation of the hand and upper extremity,* 5th ed. St. Louis, Mosby, 2002.)

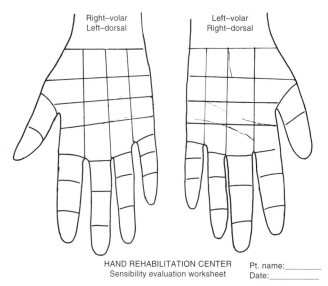

Right–volar
Left–dorsal

Left–volar
Right–dorsal

HAND REHABILITATION CENTER
Sensibility evaluation worksheet

Pt. name:_____
Date:_____

FIGURE 3-73 Hand grid worksheet. (From Callahan AD: Sensibility assessment for nerve lesions-in-continuity and nerve lacerations. In Skirven TM, Osterman AL, Fedorczyk J, et al (eds): *Rehabilitation of the hand and upper extremity,* 5th ed. St. Louis, Mosby, 2002.)

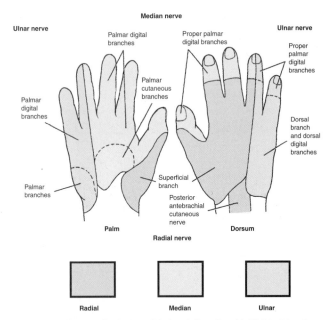

FIGURE 3-74 Sensory distribution of the hand. (From Trumble TE: *Principles of hand surgery and therapy*. Philadelphia, WB Saunders, 2000, p 14.)

Pain Sensation

Pain is an unpleasant sensory and perceptual experience associated with actual or potential cellular damage. The experience of pain is subjective and multidimensional. Pain can be tested by pinching the digit firmly or by pinprick. Intact pain sensation is indicative of protective sensation. The pinprick test can be used to rule out a digital nerve laceration. Be sure to use universal precautions.

TEST FOR PAIN (PROTECTIVE SENSATION)

Procedure

- Using a sterilized safety pin, assess the amount of pressure required to elicit a pain response on the uninvolved hand. This is

the amount of pressure that the examiner will use on the involved side.
- Alternate randomly between the sharp and dull sides of the safety pin, ensuring that each spot has one sharp and one dull application (Fig. 3-75).

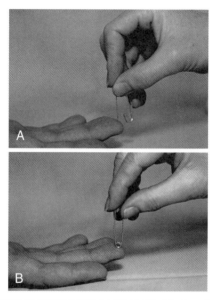

FIGURE 3-75 Sensory testing for sharp and dull. **A,** sharp, **B,** dull.

Response
- The client indicates "sharp" or "dull" following application.

Scoring
- The correct response to both sharp and dull indicates intact protective sensation.
- The incorrect response to both sharp and dull indicates absent protective sensation.

Temperature Awareness

Temperature awareness is a test for protective sensation. Thermal receptors detect warmth and cold. In the clinic, it is important to test temperature sensation prior to applying heat or cold modalities to avoid burn injuries. Thermal receptors are also critical for a person to be able to determine safe water temperature for bathing. The client who lacks temperature awareness must learn compensatory strategies such as testing water temperature with an unaffected body part. Many clinicians use only the pinprick test as sufficient evidence of protective sensation.

TEST FOR TEMPERATURE AWARENESS (PROTECTIVE SENSATION)

Procedure
- Using test tubes or metal cylinders filled with hot or cold fluid, apply randomly to areas of the involved hand (Fig. 3-76).

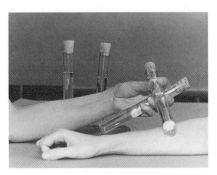

FIGURE 3-76 Test for temperature awareness.

Response
- The client indicates "hot" or "cold" following application.

Scoring
- The correct response to both cold and hot indicates intact temperature awareness.
- The incorrect response to either or both indicates impaired temperature awareness.

Testing for Touch Sensation

TWO-POINT DISCRIMINATION

Two-point discrimination and touch pressure using monofilaments are tests of different aspects of sensation. Two-point discrimination is a test for receptor density and is a good test to use for mapping improvement following nerve repair. Moving two-point discrimination returns before static two-point discrimination and is an indicator of recovery; it is typically noticed before static two-point discrimination improves.

TEST FOR STATIC TWO-POINT DISCRIMINATION

Procedure

- Use a device such as the Disk-Criminator (AliMed, Dedham, Mass.) or Boley Gauge (Integra, Plainsboro, NJ) with blunt testing ends (Fig. 3-77).

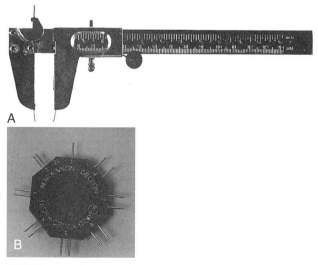

FIGURE 3-77 A, Boley gauge. **B,** Disk-Criminator for testing static and moving two-point discrimination.

- Test only the fingertips, because this is the primary area of the hand used in exploration of objects.
- Begin with 5 mm of distance between the testing points.
- Randomly apply one or two points on the radial and ulnar aspects of each finger for 10 applications (Fig. 3-78).

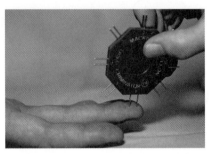

FIGURE 3-78 Two-point discrimination testing

- The pressure applied is light; stop just when the skin begins to blanch.

Response
- The client will respond "one" or "two," or "I don't know," following application.

Scoring
- The client responds accurately to seven out of ten applications at that number of millimeters of distance between the two points.
- Norms are as follows:
  - 1-5 mm indicates normal static two-point discrimination.
  - 6-10 mm indicates fair static two-point discrimination.
  - 11-15 mm indicates poor static two-point discrimination.
  - One point perceived indicates protective sensation only.
  - No points perceived indicates anesthetic area.

TEST FOR MOVING TWO-POINT DISCRIMINATION
Procedure
- Begin with a distance of 8 mm between points.
- Randomly select one or two points and move proximal to distal on the distal phalanx parallel to the longitudinal axis of the

finger, so as to not stimulate the adjacent digital nerve (see Fig. 3-78).
- The pressure applied is just enough for the client to appreciate the stimulus.
- If the client responds accurately, decrease the distance between the points and repeat the sequence until you find the smallest distance that the client can accurately perceive.

Response
- Client states "one," "two," or "I don't know."

Scoring
- The client responds accurately to seven out of ten applications.
- Norms are as follows:
  - 2-4 mm for ages 4 to 60 years indicates normal moving two-point discrimination.
  - 4-6 mm for ages 60 years and older indicates normal moving two-point discrimination.

Touch Pressure

Light touch is perceived by receptors in the superficial skin. Pressure (or deeper touch) is perceived by receptors in subcutaneous and deeper tissues. Although light touch is important for fine discriminatory hand use, deep pressure is important as a form of protective sensation. Touch pressure testing examines the spectrum from light touch to deep pressure. Touch pressure testing is a good test to use for clients with nerve entrapments, such as carpal tunnel syndrome.

Touch pressure is tested with a set of 20 monofilaments. These monofilaments are of varying thicknesses, with numbers that represent a mathematical formula of the force required to bow them when applied perpendicularly. They are color-coded to correspond to five threshold categories. Clinicians will frequently use an abbreviated set of five monofilaments, one for each of these categories.

TEST FOR TOUCH PRESSURE

Procedure
- Begin with monofilament 1.65.
- Apply the monofilament in 1 to 1.5 seconds using the pressure needed to bow the monofilament (applied with a perpendicular position; Fig. 3-79).

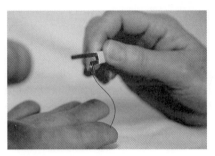

FIGURE 3-79 Application of touch pressure monofilament to client's fingertip.

- Hold the pressure for 1 to 1.5 seconds.
- Lift the monofilament in 1 to 1.5 seconds.
- The proper amount of pressure is achieved when the filament bends.
- Repeat this three times in the same spot for monofilaments 1.65 to 4.08; monofilaments higher than 4.08 are applied only once.
- Randomly select areas of the hand to test and change the interval of time between the applications of monofilaments.
- If the client does not perceive the monofilament, proceed to the next (thicker) monofilament and repeat the sequence until monofilament 6.65.
- If client does perceive the monofilament, record this number on the hand grid and proceed to the next area of the hand.

Response
- Client says "touch" when he or she feels the monofilament.

Scoring
- The client responds to at least one of the three applications of the monofilament.
- Norms are as follows:
  - Green (1.65 to 2.83) indicates normal light touch.
  - Blue (3.22 to 3.61) indicates diminished light touch.
  - Purple (3.84 to 4.31) indicates diminished protective sensation.
  - Red (4.56 to 6.65) indicates loss of protective sensation.
  - Untestable indicates inability to feel the largest monofilament.

Proprioception

Conscious proprioception derives from receptors found in the muscles, tendons, and joints and is defined as the awareness of joint position in space. It is through cerebral integration of information about touch and proprioception that objects can be identified by tactile cues and pressure. If proprioception is impaired, it may be difficult to gauge how much pressure to use when holding a paper cup.

TEST FOR PROPRIOCEPTION

Procedure
- Hold the lateral aspects of the elbow, wrist, or digit.
- Move the body part in flexion or extension (Fig. 3-80).

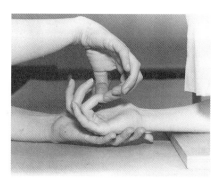

FIGURE 3-80 Testing proprioception of the finger.

Response
- Client indicates if the body part is being moved "up" or "down."

Scoring
- Accurate response indicates intact proprioception.

The term *kinesthesia* is sometimes used interchangeably with the term *proprioception* but can also be defined as awareness of joint movement. Some therapists make a distinction between these two terms, testing for kinesthesia by moving the unaffected limb into a certain posture and having the client copy the movement with the affected side while her or his eyes are closed.

Stereognosis

Stereognosis is the use of proprioceptive information and touch information to identify an item with vision occluded. Without stereognosis, it is impossible to pick out a specific object such as a coin or a key from one's pocket, or use a zipper that fastens behind you, or pick up a plate from a sink of sudsy water.

The Dellon modification of the Moberg Pickup Test is a good test for stereognosis for clients with injuries involving the median and/or ulnar nerves. This test requires the client's ability to participate motorically, so motor loss or weakness should be factored in to the choice of this assessment. This test is based on the Moberg Pickup Test, which is a timed motor test that does not require object identification.

DELLON MODIFICATION OF THE MOBERG PICKUP TEST

Procedure

- Begin with a group of 12 standardized items: wing nut, large nut, hex nut, small square nut, screw, key, nickel, dime, washer, safety pin, paper clip, and nail.
- If the ulnar nerve is not involved, tape the ulnar two fingers to the client's palm if possible.

Test 1

- The client places the items one at a time into a box as quickly as possible.
- Record the time for two trials.

Test 2. Initiate test 2 only if the client's deficits do not appear too severe during test 1.

- With the client's vision occluded, the examiner places the items into the client's radial three digits one at a time.
- The examiner records the time that it takes to identify each item, with a maximum of 30 seconds for each item.
- Each item is placed in the client's hand twice.

Response

- Test 1: The client places items in a box using radial three digits as quickly as possible.
- Test 2: The client manipulates objects and attempts to identify them as quickly as possible.

Scoring
- Test 1: The time it takes to place all items in the box
- Test 2: The time it takes to identify all the items

Localization of Touch

Localization of touch is considered to be a test of functional sensation because there is a high correlation between this test and the test for two-point discrimination. Localization of touch is an important test to perform following nerve repair because it helps determine the client's baseline and projected functional prognosis. This test can be done with a constant (static) touch or a moving touch. Localization of touch is thought by many to reflect a cognitive component of the client's abilities. Because it is considered to be a test of tactile discrimination that requires cortical processing, it is different from touch pressure testing.

TEST FOR LOCALIZATION OF TOUCH

Procedure
- Apply the finest monofilament that the client can perceive to the center of a corresponding zone on the hand grid.
- Once the client feels a touch, have him or her open the eyes and use the index finger to point to the exact area where the stimulus was felt.
- Place a dot on the hand grid for a correct response.
- Place an arrow from the site of the actual stimulation to the identified site if the stimulus is incorrectly identified.

Response
- The client attempts to identify the exact location of a stimulus.

Scoring
The correct identification of area within 1 cm of actual placement indicates intact touch localization.

Desensitization uses graded stimulation with procedures and modalities that are slightly aversive but tolerable. The stimuli are upgraded to be slightly more noxious as the client's tolerance increases. The client's hand is exposed to textures such as sandpaper and contact particles such as rice, and vibration. Treatment is done for 10-minute intervals, three or four times a day.

PROTECTIVE SENSORY REEDUCATION

- Protect from being exposed to sharp items or to cold or heat.
- Try to soften the amount of force used when gripping an object.
- Use built-up handles on objects whenever possible to distribute gripping pressure over a greater surface area.
- Do not persist in an activity for prolonged periods. Instead, change the tool used and rotate the work task often.
- Visually examine the skin for edema, redness, warmth, blisters, cuts, or other wounds. This is important because tissue heals more slowly when there has been a nerve injury.
- If there is tissue injury or damage, be very careful in treating, and try to avoid infection.
- Maintain skin suppleness as much as possible by applying moisturizing agents.

DISCRIMINATIVE SENSORY REEDUCATION

Localization

Localization of moving touch tends to return before localization of constant touch. Retraining is done for both. With the client's eyes closed, the eraser end of a pencil or the therapist's finger is touched to the client's hand in the midline of one zone of the hand grid. This makes the documentation easier and the intervention more accurate and consistent, and minimizes afferent activity from adjacent areas of the skin. The stimulus is applied with a moving or constant touch. The client is told to open his or her eyes and point to the area that was touched.

Graded Discrimination

Stimulation is graded from that requiring gross discrimination to that requiring fine discrimination. Levels of difficulty in discrimination are represented by the sequencing of these three categories: (1) same or different; (2) how they are the same or different; and (3) identification of the material or object.

Another version of discriminative training involves tracing a geometric shape, letter, or number on the fingertip or small area of the hand. This can be applied with a fingertip or the end of an instrument such as a small dowel or a pencil eraser. The client tries to identify the figure.

Evaluation and Treatment of Visual Deficits Following Brain Injury

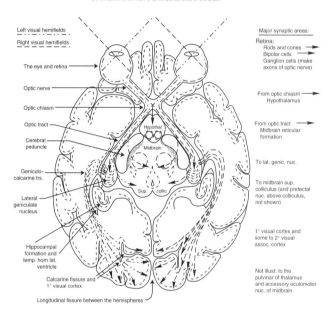

PARALLEL-DISTRIBUTED PROCESSING OF THE VISUAL SYSTEM-I

Schematic inferior view of a horizontal slice of the brain

Left visual hemifields

Right visual hemifields

The eye and retina

Optic nerve

Optic chiasm

Optic tract

Cerebral peduncle

Geniculo-calcarine trs.

Lateral geniculate nucleus

Hippocampal formation and temp. horn lat. ventricle

Calcarine fissure and 1° visual cortex

Longitudinal fissure between the hemispheres

Hypothal.

Midbrain

Sup. collic.

Major synaptic areas:

Retina:
  Rods and cones
  Bipolar cells
  Ganglion cells (make axons of optic nerve)

From optic chiasm
  Hypothalamus

From optic tract
  Midbrain reticular formation

To lat. genic. nuc.

To midbrain sup. colliculus (and pretectal nuc. above colliculus, not shown)

1° visual cortex and some to 2° visual assoc. cortex

Not illust: to the pulvinar of thalamus and accessory oculomotor nuc. of midbrain

The visual system is our most important sense in regard to:

A. Learning, memory, and recall including our ability to see color and fine details as well as the visual surround and global relationships.
B. Communication: use of symbolic language, speaking, and body language.
C. Spatiotemporal orientation in concert with vestibular-proprioceptive systems.
D. Early warning system to pleasure or danger, i.e., vision is our farthest reaching distance receptor and movement detector par excellence.
E. Visual-manual and visual-motor activities.

1°, Primary.
2°, Secondary.

FIGURE 3-81 Pathways from retina to LGN to visual cortex. (Courtesy of Dr. Josephine C. Moore.)

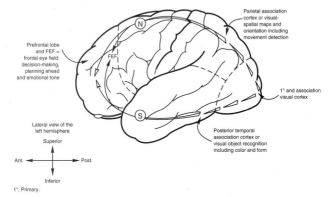

PARALLEL-DISTRIBUTED PROCESSING OF THE VISUAL SYSTEM

Two parallel routes carry visual information from the occipital lobe to the prefrontal lobe and frontal eye field (FEF). Fibers from these two routes distribute to many areas along each route (not illustrated) before terminating in the prefrontal cortex and FEF as illustrated.

(N) = "Northern" or superior route via parietal and frontal lobes.

(S) = "Southern" or inferior route via temporal and frontal lobes.

Parietal association cortex or visual-spatial maps and orientation including movement detection

Prefrontal lobe and FEF = frontal eye field: decision-making, planning ahead and emotional tone

1° and association visual cortex

Lateral view of the left hemisphere

Superior

Ant. ◄────► Post.

Inferior

Posterior temporal association cortex or visual object recognition including color and form

1°, Primary.

FIGURE 3-82 Visual input travels from the visual cortex through parietal and posterior temporal circuitry to the prefrontal lobe to complete cortical visual processing. (Courtesy of Dr. Josephine C. Moore.)

TABLE 3-4 Summary of Cortical Hemispheric Functions for Visual Processing and Deficits Secondary to Lesion Site

Left Hemisphere Advantage		Right Hemisphere Advantage	
More detail-oriented in relation to persons, places, and things; takes in minute details and compares and contrasts these details; processes visual information sequentially in a systematic item by item, serial search strategy; attends only to right visual fields		More global or holistic; takes a general view of the environment; processes multiple visual inputs simultaneously, grouping them into meaningful categories; attends globally to left and right visual fields	
Parietal Lesion	Posterior Temporal Lesion	Parietal Lesion	Posterior Tempotal Lesion
Biases attention to detail	Biases attention to global input	Biases attention to detail	Biases attention to global input
Biases brain to right advantages	Biases brain to right hemisphere advantages	Biases brain to left hemisphere advantages	Biases brain to left hemisphere advantages
May have right inferior quadrant visual field loss	May have right superior quadrant visual field loss	May have neglect or hemi-inattention along with left inferior quadrant visual field loss	May have neglect or hemi-inattention along with left superior quadrant visual field loss

Adapted with permission of Dr. Josephine C. Moore.

Intervention

- Increase background contrast.
- Increase illumination.
- Reduce background pattern.
- Enlarge objects or features that need to be seen.
- Organize.
- Access community services.

TABLE 3-5 Comparison of Search Patterns Between Persons with Visual Field Deficit and Persons with Hemi-Inattention

Visual Field Deficit	Hemi-Inattention
Search pattern is abbreviated toward blind field	Search pattern is asymmetrical; initiated or confined to the right side
Attempts to direct search toward blind side	No attempt to direct search toward left side
Search pattern is organized and generally efficient	Search pattern is random and generally inefficient
Client rescans to check accuracy of performance	Client does not rescan to check accuracy of performance
Time spent on task is appropriate to level of difficulty	Client completes task quickly; level of effort applied not consistent with difficulty of task

Adapted from Warren M: *Brain injury visual assessment battery for adults test manual.* Lenexa, Kan, visAbilities Rehab Services, 1998.

TABLE 3-6 Summary of Oculomotor Deficits Associated with Cranial Nerve Lesions

Oculomotor Nerve III	Trochlear Nerve IV	Abducens Nerve VI
Impaired vertical eye movements	Impaired downward and lateral eye movements	Impaired lateral eye movements
Lateral diplopia for near vision tasks	Vertical diplopia for near vision tasks	Lateral diplopia for far vision tasks
Dilation of pupil and impaired accommodation	With bilateral lesion, assumes downward head tilt	
Ptosis of eyelid		

Assessment and Intervention for Perceptual Dysfunction

TABLE 3-7 Elements of Comprehensive Apraxia Assessment

Test Condition	Example
Gesture to command	"Show me how you would take off your hat." (transitive) "Show me how you would throw a kiss." (intransitive)
Gesture to imitation	"Copy what I do." Therapist shrugs shoulders. (intransitive) Therapist flips an imaginary coin. (transitive)
Gesture in response to seeing the tool	"Show me how you would seeing the tool use this object." Therapist provides screwdriver for display.
Gesture in response to seeing the object upon which the tool works	"Show me how you would use this object." Therapist provides screwdriver and block of wood with screw partially inserted.
Actual tool use	"Show me how you would use this object." Therapist provides screwdriver for use.
Imitation of the examiner using the tool	"Copy what I do." Therapist makes stirring motion, using a spoon.
Discrimination between correct and incorrect pantomimed movements	"Is this the correct way to blow out a match?" Therapist pantomimes holding a match in an unsafe manner (e.g., match held upside down, with the head of the match near the palm of hand).
Gesture comprehension	"What object am I using?" Therapist pantomimes by shaving face with a razor.
Serial acts	"Show me how you would open an imaginary can of soda, pour it into a glass, and take a drink."

From Heilman KM, Rothi LJG: Apraxia. In Heilman KM, Valenstein E (eds): *Clinical neuropsychology*, New York, Oxford University Press, 1993, pp.

Evaluation and Treatment of Limited Occupational Performance Secondary to Cognitive Dysfunction

TABLE 3-8 Instruments to Document Improved Function in Those with Functional Limitations Secondary to Presence of Cognitive Impairments

Instrument	Description
Standardized, valid, and reliable measures of quality of life	Measures life satisfaction and well-being (e.g., Medical Outcomes Study, 36-item Short-Form Health Survey, World Health Organization Quality of Life Scale, Reintegration to Normal Living); see text for details.
Standardized, valid, and reliable measures of areas of occupation (e.g., BADL, IADL, leisure, work)	Measures performance in areas of occupation (e.g., Functional Independence Measure, Barthel Index, Lawton Instrumental Activities of Daily Living Scale); see text for details.
Standardized, valid, and reliable measures of participation	Measures involvement in life situations (e.g., Activity Card Sort, Community Integration Questionnaire, and the Canadian Occupational Performance Measure); see text for details.
Comprehensive Measures*	
Árnadóttir OT-ADL Neurobehavioral Evaluation[†]	Performance-based tool that uses structured observations of upper and lower body dressing, grooming, hygiene, feeding, transfers, mobility and communication to detect the underlying impairments that interfere with function (e.g., impairments include decreased organization and sequencing, short- and long-term memory loss, decreased alertness and arousal, impaired attention, performance latency, confusion, perseveration, distractibility, impaired initiation, insight, judgment)
Assessment of Motor and Process Skills (AMPS)	Client-centered performance assessment of BADL and IADL, with an emphasis placed on IADL tasks. The AMPS involves the client choosing to perform two or three tasks in collaboration with a therapist from a list of more than 80 standardized tasks. It evaluates motor and processing skills that affect function. Process skills are observable actions that a person uses to to do the following: (1) select, interact with, and use tools and materials; (2) carry out individual actions and steps; and (3) modify performance when problems are encountered. Process skills should not be confused with cognitive skills.
Brief Measure of Cognitive Functional Performance	
Kettle Test	Provides a brief performance-based assessment of an IADL task designed to tap into a broad range of cognitive skills. The task consists of making two hot beverages that differ in two ingredients (one for the client and one for the therapist). The electric kettle is emptied and disassembled to challenge problem-solving, safety, and judgment skills; additional kitchen utensils and ingredients are placed as distracters to increase attention demands.

TABLE 3-8 Instruments to Document Improved Function in Those with Functional Limitations Secondary to Presence of Cognitive Impairments—cont'd

Instrument	Description
Assessing Executive Function Impairments	
Executive Function Performance Test (EFPT)	Assesses executive function deficits during the performance of real-world tasks (e.g., cooking oatmeal, making a phone call, managing medications, paying a bill). The test uses a structured cueing and scoring system to assess initiation, organization, safety, and task completion and develop cueing strategies.
Calendar Planning Test	This calendar planning activity is a higher level simulated IADL task that involves entering 17 appointments and errands into a weekly schedule. It was designed to be sensitive to the effects of executive dysfunction because it requires planning, organization, and multitasking abilities. In addition to entering appointments, the person must monitor time, keep track of rules, inhibit distractions, and deal with schedule conflicts.
Multiple Errands Test	Multitasking assessment that challenges multiple executive functions. Tasks include purchasing three items, picking up an envelope from reception, using the telephone, sending the envelope, writing down four items (e.g., price of a candy bar), meeting assessor, and informing assessor that the test was completed.
Executive Function Route Finding Task	Uses naturalistic observations of route finding to detect dysexecutive symptoms
Behavioural Assessment of the Dysexecutive Syndrome (BADS)	Battery designed to assess capabilities that are typically required in everyday living. It includes six subtests that represent different executive abilities (e.g., cognitive flexibility, novel problem solving, planning, judgment and estimation, behavioral regulation). It uses simulated everyday tasks.
Assessing Memory Loss	
Rivermead Behavioral Memory Test, 3rd Edition	Ecologically valid test of everyday memory; Uues simulations of everyday memory tasks. Modifications are available for those with perceptual, language, and mobility impairments.
Cambridge Behavioural Prospective Memory Test, Cambridge Prospective Memory Test	Objective test of prospective memory
Assessing Impairments of Attention	
Test of Everyday Attention	Considered an ecologically valid test of various types of everyday attention (e.g., sustained attention, selective attention, attentional switching, divided attention). Includes several subtests. It is one of the few tests of attention that simulates everyday life tasks. The test is based on the imagined scenario of a vacation trip to the Philadelphia area.

Continued

TABLE 3-8 Instruments to Document Improved Function in Those with Functional Limitations Secondary to Presence of Cognitive Impairments—cont'd

Instrument	Description
Moss Attention Rating Scale	Observational test of disordered attention (22-item version); produces three factor scores and a total score
Rating Scale of Attentional Behaviour	Short assessment of attention-based impairments rated via clinicians' observations of behaviors

BADL, Basic ADL.
*These simultaneously assess activity and/or participation and underlying impairments or subskills.
†More recently referred to as the ADL-Focused Occupation-Based Neurobehavioral Evaluation (A-ONE)

TABLE 3-9 Examples of Self and/or Caregiver Report Measures

Instrument	Instrument Description
Attention Rating and Monitoring Scale	Self-report measure of the frequency of everyday problems related to attention impairments
Cognitive Failures Questionnaire	Self-report measure of the frequency of lapses of attention and cognition in daily life; Includes items related to memory, attention, and executive dysfunction
Prospective Memory Questionnaire	Behaviorally anchored self-rated evaluation of prospective memory.
Comprehensive Assessment of Prospective Memory	Assessment of prospective memory related to BADL and IADL
Everyday Memory Questionnaire	Subjective report of everyday memory; metamemory questionnaire; Self-report or via proxy
Prospective and Retrospective Memory Questionnaire	Measure of prospective and retrospective failures in everyday life; Self-rated or proxy-rated. Norms are published.
Dysexecutive Questionnaire*	20-item questionnaire sampling everyday symptoms associated with executive functions impairments. Versions with self-rating and ratings by significant others* are available.
Behavior Rating Inventory of Executive Function, Adult Version	Documents adult's executive functions or self-regulation in the everyday environment; includes a self-report and an informant report

Part of the BADS test battery; see Table 3-9.

TABLE 3-10 Examples of Standardized Tests of Awareness

Instrument	Brief Description
Self-Awareness of Deficits Interview	This is an interviewer-rated structured interview used to obtain quantitative and qualitative data on the status of self-awareness after brain injury. Specifically, it assesses a client's level of intellectual awareness (the ability to understand that a function is decreased from the premorbid level and to recognize implications of deficits).
Self-Regulation Skills Interview	This is a semistructured clinician-rated interview. The tool includes six questions that assess metacognitive or self-regulation skills.
Patient Competency Rating Scale (PCRS)	This tool evaluates self-awareness following a TBI. It is a 30-item, self-report instrument that uses a five-point Likert scale (1 = can't do and 5 = can do with ease) to self-rate the degree of difficulty in a variety of tasks and functions. A modified yet still psychometrically sound version of the PCRS was developed for use on an acute, inpatient neurorehabilitation unit. This version retained 13 items from the original PCRS.
Awareness Questionnaire	This is a measure of impaired self-awareness after a TBI. The instrument consists of three forms (one form is completed by the client, one by a significant other, and one by a clinician). The self-rated and family's or significant others' forms contain 17 items and the clinician's form contains 18 items. The client's abilities to perform various tasks after the injury as compared with before the injury are rated on a five-point scale.
Awareness Interview	This tool is used to evaluate awareness of cognitive and motor defects after cerebral infarction, dementia, or head trauma. Operationally, the authors defined unawareness as a discrepancy between the client's opinion of his or her abilities in the interview and his or her abilities as measured in neuropsychological and neurologic examinations.
Assessment of Awareness of Disability	This is an assessment based on a semistructured interview, which is used in conjunction with the Assessment of Motor and Process Skills (AMPS). It consists of general and specific questions related to ADL tasks; the interview is conducted after performance of the AMPS.

TABLE 3-11 Prompting Procedures to Promote Awareness of Errors During Functional Activities

Prompt	Rationale
"How do you know this is the right answer or procedure?" or "Tell me why you chose this answer/procedure."	Refocuses client's attention to task performance and error detection. Can client self-correct with a general cue?
"That is not correct. Can you see why?"	Provides general feedback about error but is not specific. Can client find error and initiate correction?
"It is not correct because . . . "	Provides specific feedback about error. Can client correct error when it is pointed out?
"Try this [strategy]" (e.g., going slower, saying each step out loud, verbalizing a plan before starting, using a checklist).	Provides client with a specific, alternate approach. Can client use strategy given?
Task is altered. "Try it another way."	Modifies task by one parameter. Can client perform task? Begin again with grading of prompting described earlier.

From Brockmann-Rubio K, Gillen G: Treatment of cognitive-perceptual impairments: A function-based approach. In Gillen G, Burkhardt A (eds): Stroke rehabilitation: A function-based approach, 2nd ed. St Louis, Elsevier/Mosby, 2004, pp 427-446.

BOX 3-4 Other Suggestions for Improving Awareness

Have clients perform tasks of interest and then provide them with feedback about their performance. The goal is to have clients monitor and observe their behavior more accurately so that they can make more realistic predictions about future performance as well gain insight into their strengths and weaknesses.

Encourage self-questioning during a task and self-evaluation after a task (e.g., "Have I completed all the steps needed?").

Provide methods of comparing functioning pre- and postinjury to improve awareness.

Use prediction methods. Have the client estimate various task parameters such as difficulty, time needed for completion, number of errors, and/or amount assistance needed before, during, or after a task and compare with actual results.

Help clients develop and appropriately set their personal goals.

Allow clients to observe their own performance during specific tasks (e.g., via videotape) and compare their actual performance to what they state they can do.

Group treatments and peer feedback may be used because one person can receive feedback on performance from multiple individuals.

Use role reversals. Have the therapist perform the task and make errors, and have the client detect the errors.

The development of a strong therapeutic alliance is critical in managing denial and lack of self-awareness. This alliance should be open and based on trust. Coaching clients to make better choices and understand how defensive strategies affect daily function.

Use familiar tasks that are graded to match the person's cognitive level ("just the right challenge") to develop self-monitoring skills and error recognition.

Provide education related to deficit areas for clients as well as families.

Integrate experiential feedback experiences. This method has been called supported risk taking and planned failures and is used during daily activities to demonstrate impairments gently. High levels of therapist supported are mandatory during this intervention.

Monitor for increased signs of depression and anxiety as awareness increases.

Increase mastery and control during performance of daily tasks to increase awareness.

Use emotionally neutral tasks to increase error recognition.

Use tasks that offer "just the right challenge" to increase error recognition/correction.

Provide feedback in a sandwich format (negative comments are preceded and followed by positive feedback).

Adapted from Gillen G: Cognitive and perceptual rehabilitation: Optimizing function, St. Louis, Elsevier/Mosby, 2009.

TABLE 3-12 Terminology Related to Attention Impairments

Attention Component	Definition	Functional Examples
Attention	Voluntary control over more automatic brain systems so as to be able to select and manipulate sensory and stored information briefly or for sustained periods	See later for examples of the specific components of attention.
Arousal	A state of responsiveness to sensory stimulation or excitability; dependent on a widely distributed neural network, including prefrontal areas and neurotransmitter systems	Decreased responsiveness to incoming visual, auditory, or tactile cues during task performance; requires noxious or extreme sensory stimuli (e.g., cold washcloth applied to the face) to elicit behavioral response
Selective attention	Type of attention involved in processing and filtering of relevant information in the presence of irrelevant stimuli; efficiency with which people can search and focus on specific information while ignoring distracters. Because selective attention is critical for encoding information into memory, retaining and manipulating information in working memory, and successfully executing goal-directed behavior, a deficit in selective attention could contribute to the numerous cognitive deficits observed in those living with neurologic impairments. This skill is linked to prefrontal and underlying anterior cingulated areas	Attending to one conversation during a party; studying outside with the noise of traffic and children playing; attending to a therapist's instructions and cues in a crowded therapy clinic; making dinner while the children are watching TV in the background; attending to a board game during recess
Sustained attention (vigilance)	Used to support tasks that require vigilance and the capacity to maintain attention over time; this construct is often measured by time spent on task. In adults, this attention component is linked to prefrontal function in the right hemisphere and white matter damage.	Being able to attend to long conversations, instructions, class lessons, television shows, or movies; attending to playing a game of chess; balancing a checkbook; watching your child on the playground

Continued

TABLE 3-12 Terminology Related to Attention Impairments—cont'd

Attention Component	Definition	Functional Examples
Attentional switching or alternating attention	The ability to switch attention flexibility from one concept to another; related to cognitive flexibility; ability to change attentive focus in a flexible or adaptive manner; ability to move between tasks with different cognitive requirements. This skill appears to be a function of the prefrontal cortex and posterior parietal lobe, thalamus, and midbrain.	While typing a paper, a friend comes into your room to discuss a completely different topic; when the conversation is over, you return to typing; Cooking, taking care of a crying child, then returning to cooking; a unit clerk at the hospital alternating between flagging orders on the medical chart, answering the phone, and writing down phone messages
Divided attention	Dividing attention between two or more tasks simultaneously; dual tasking or multitasking; ability to attend to two competing stimuli simultaneously. Deficits occur when limited attentional resources are divided between two sources.	Making toast and tea at the same time; texting while carrying on a conversation; playing cards while discussing the events of the day
Distractibility	Breakdown in selective attention; inability to block out environmental or internal stimuli when one is trying to concentrate on performing a particular task; symptom of prefrontal damage, particularly the dorsolateral cortex	Noise in the hallway takes away your attention while taking notes during a class; inability to attend during a therapy session because of being distracted by watching someone else's session
Field-dependent behavior	Distracted by and acting on an irrelevant impulse that interferes with activity performance and takes over goal-directed activity; includes both an attention and perseveration component	While performing oral care, a person becomes distracted by a light switch; the person then stops the oral care activity while turning on and off the light switch (i.e., not relevant to the task at hand).
Unilateral neglect (a lateralized attention deficit)	See chapter - your chapter on CVA	See chapter – your chapter on CVA

Adapted from Gillen G: *Cognitive and perceptual rehabilitation: optimizing function.* St. Louis, Elsevier/Mosby, 2009.

BOX 3-5 Managing Attention Deficits: Strategies for Clinicians and Caretakers

Avoid overstimulating or distracting environments.
> Face away from visual distracters during tasks.
> Wear earplugs.
> Shop or go to restaurants at off-peak times.
> Use filing systems to enhance organization.
> Label cupboards and drawers.
> Reduce clutter and visual distracters.
> Use self-instruction strategies.
> Use time pressure management strategies.
> Teach self-pacing strategies.
> Control the rate of incoming information.
> Self-manage effort and emotional responses during tasks.
> Teach monitoring or shared attentional resources when multitasking.
> Manage the home environment to decrease auditory and visual stimuli. Keep radios and phones turned off. Close doors and curtains. Keep surfaces, cabinets, closets, and refrigerators organized and uncluttered.
> Use daily checklists for work, self-care, and instrumental activities of daily living.

Adapted from Gillen G: *Cognitive and perceptual rehabilitation: Optimizing function.* St. Louis, Elsevier/Mosby, 2009.

TABLE 3-13 Terminology Related to Memory Impairments

Term	Definition	Examples of Everyday Behaviors
Anterograde amnesia	A deficit in new learning; an inability to recall information learned after acquired brain damage; an inability to form new memories after brain damage occurs	Not able to recall staff names, easily gets lost secondary to topographic disorientation, not able to recall what occurred in therapy this morning; difficulty learning adaptive strategies to compensate for memory loss
Retrograde amnesia	Difficulty recalling memories formed and stored prior to the disease onset; may be worse for recent events as opposed to substantially older memories	Inability to remember autobiographic information (e.g., address, social security number, birth order), historical events (e.g., war, presidential elections, scientific breakthroughs), and/or personally experienced events (e.g., weddings, vacations)
Short-term memory	Storage of limited information for a limited amount of time	Difficulty remembering instructions related to the use of adaptive equipment; not able to remember the names of someone just introduced at a dinner party; not able to remember "today's specials" in a restaurant
Working memory	Related to short-term memory; refers to actively manipulating information that is in short-term storage via rehearsals	While playing a board game, unable to remember and use the rules of the game; not able to perform calculations mentally while balancing the checkbook; difficulty remembering and adapting a recipe
Long-term memory (LTM)	Relatively permanent storing of information with unlimited capacity	May affect declarative memory of knowledge, episodes, and facts or nondeclarative memories (e.g., those related to skills and habits)

Continued

TABLE 3-13 Terminology Related to Memory Impairments—cont'd

Term	Definition	Examples of Everyday Behaviors
Nondeclarative or implicit or procedural memory	Knowing how to perform a skill, retaining previously learned skills and learning new skills; form of LTM	Driving, playing sports, making hand crafts, learning to use adaptive ADL equipment or wheelchair
Declarative or explicit memory	Knowing that something was learned, verbal retrieval of a knowledge base such as facts, and remembering everyday events; includes episodic and semantic information; form of LTM (see following)	See episodic and semantic memory.
Episodic memory	Autobiographic memory for contextually specific events; personally experienced events; form of declarative LTM	Remembering the day's events, what one had for breakfast, occurrences on the job, content of therapy sessions
Semantic memory	Knowledge of the general world, facts, linguistic skill, and vocabulary (**NOTE:** may be spared after injury); form of declarative LTM	Remembering the dates of holidays, name of the president, dates of world events
Explicit memory	Consists of memories from events that have occurred in the external world. Information stored in explicit memory is about a specific event that happened at a specific time and place.	Remembering places and names, and various words. See declarative memory.
Implicit memory	Does not require conscious retrieval of the past; knowledge is expressed in performance without the person being aware of possessing this knowledge; consists of memories necessary to perform events and tasks or produce a specific type of response	Memory of skills, habits, and subconscious processes. See nondeclarative memory.
Prospective memory	Remembering to carry out future intentions	Remembering to take medications, return phone calls, buy food, pick up children from school, mail the bills; a critical aspect of memory to support everyday living
Metamemory	Awareness of your own memory abilities	Knowing when you need to compensate for memory capacity (e.g., making a list of errands, shopping list, writing down a new phone number or driving directions, recognizing errors in memory)

Adapted From Gillen G: *Cognitive and perceptual rehabilitation: Optimizing function.* St. Louis, Elsevier/Mosby, 2009.

TABLE 3-14   Stages of Memory

Stage of Memory	Description	Neuroanatomic Area of Function
Attention	Processes that allow a person to gain access to and use incoming information; inclusive of alertness, arousal, and various attention processes such as selective attention	Brainstem; thalamic structures; frontal lobes
Encoding	How memories are formed; an initial stage of memory that analyzes the material to be remembered (visual versus verbal characteristics of information). Correct analysis of information is required for proper storage of the information.	Dorsomedial thalamus; frontal lobes; language system (e.g., Wernicke's area); visual system (e.g., visual association areas)
Storage	How memories are retained; transfer of a transient memory to a form or location in the brain for permanent retention or access	Hippocampus; bilateral medial temporal lobes
Retrieval	How memories are recalled; searching for or activating existing memory traces	Frontal lobe

Data from Sohlberg MM, Mateer CA: Memory theory applied to intervention. In Sohlberg MM, Mateer CA (eds): *Cognitive rehabilitation: An integrative neuropsychological approach.* New York, Guilford Press, 2001, pp 162-193.

BOX 3-6   Suggestions for Working with Those with Working Memory Deficits

Shorten the length of directions and instructions.

Use real-world functional tasks for training (e.g., adding monthly bills as opposed to practicing rote number strings).

Avoid fast speaking rates.

Place stress on target words during training to help the person realize the key part of the instruction. In addition, place key information at the beginning and end of sentences.

Increase the automaticity of responding by extra practice and rehearsal such as learning to transfer from a wheelchair to a bed.

Use part-whole learning or break the task down into components to promote overlearning of the components.

Teach rehearsal strategies.

Data from Parente R, Kolakowsky-Hayner S, Krug K, et al: Retraining working memory after traumatic brain injury, *NeuroRehabilitation* 13:157-163, 1999.

TABLE 3-15   List and Purpose of Memory Notebook Sections

Notebook Section	Purpose
Daily log	Used to record, store, and retrieve information about daily activities; contains forms for charting hourly information and scheduling appointments; contains forms for prioritizing a task list
Calendar	Used for recording appointments and retrieving information about important meetings and upcoming events
Names	Used to record, store, and retrieve identifying information and name drawings of new people
Current work	Used for recording specific procedures about work assignments that may be needed at a later date
Personal notes	Used for recording important personal information such as personal goals or autobiographic information; also used for recording notes such as addresses, birthdays

From Schmitter-Edgecombe M, Fahy JF, Whelan JP, et al: Memory remediation after severe closed head injury: Notebook training versus supportive therapy. *J Consult Clin Psychol* 63:484-489, 1995.

BOX 3-7   Assistive Technology for Those with Memory Loss

Handheld computers
Smart phones
Paging systems
Voice recorders
Personal data assistants
Alarm watches
Electronic pill box
Microwave with preset times
Adaptive stove controls to turn off an electric stove after a certain period of time or when heat becomes excessive
Phone with programmable memory buttons (affix pictures to the buttons)
Phone with buttons programmed to speak the name of the person being called
Key locator attachment
Recording used to cue a behavioral sequence such as morning care

Adapted from Gillen G: Cognitive and perceptual rehabilitation: Optimizing function, St. Louis, Elsevier/Mosby, 2009.

BOX 3-8 Strategies for Significant Others of Those Living with Memory Loss

Understand that this impairment often may not be reversible.

Become very familiar with the specific type of compensatory memory strategies that have been prescribed.

Keep daily schedules as consistent as possible; stick with habits and routines.

Simplify the environment by decreasing clutter and keeping the living areas organized.

Decrease excessive environmental stimuli.

Help by organizing calendars, clocks, and reminders posted around the house.

Be proactive in identifying potential safety issues.

Use short and direct sentences.

Make sure that the most important information comes at the beginning the sentence.

Highlight, cue, and emphasize key aspects of communication (e.g., repeat, point).

Avoid conversations that rely on memory—keep conversations in the present.

Repetition of sentences may be inevitable.

Summarize conversations.

Remember that in many cases, intelligence may remain intact.

Keep "a place for everything and everything in its place."

Use photographs, souvenirs, and other appropriate items to help access memories.

Understand that fatigue, stress, sleep disorders, and depression can exacerbate memory loss.

Keep back-up items (e.g., glasses, spare keys).

Help create to-do lists. Remind loved ones to check off or highlight the item when the task is completed.

Label items, drawers, and shelves.

Adapted from Gillen G: *Cognitive and perceptual rehabilitation: Optimizing function*, St. Louis, Elsevier/Mosby, 2009.

TABLE 3-16 Executive Functions Related to Everyday Living: Preparing a Salad

Executive Function	Associated Tasks
Initiation	Starting the task at the appropriate time without overreliance on prompts
Organization	Organizing the work space and performing the task efficiently (e.g., gathering necessary vegetables at the same time from the refrigerator)
Sequencing	Sequencing the steps of the task appropriately (e.g., gather tools and vegetables, wash vegetables, chop and slice vegetables, mix in bowl, add dressing)
Problem solving	Solving the problem of a using a knife that is too dull for slicing

From Gillen G: *Cognitive and perceptual rehabilitation: Optimizing function.* St. Louis, Elsevier/Mosby, 2009.

Eating and Swallowing

TABLE 3-17   Outer Oral Motor Assessment

Function	Instruction to Client	Testing Procedure*
Facial expression	"Lift your eyebrows as high as you can."	Place one finger above each eyebrow. Apply downward pressure.
	"Bring your eyebrows toward your nose in a frown."	Place one finger above each eyebrow. Apply pressure outward.
	"Wrinkle your nose upward."	Place one finger on tip of nose and apply downward pressure.
	"Suck in your cheeks."	Apply pressure outward against each inside cheek.
Lip control	"Smile."	Observe for symmetrical movement. Palpate over each cheek.
	"Press your lips together tightly and puff out your cheeks."	Place one finger above and one finger below lips. Apply pressure, moving fingers away from each other; check for ability to hold air.
	"Pucker your lips as in a kiss."	Apply pressure inwardly against lips (toward teeth).
Jaw control	"Open your mouth as far as you can."	Help patient maintain head control. Apply pressure from under chin upward and forward.
	"Close your mouth tightly. Don't let me open it."	Help client maintain head control. Apply pressure on chin downward.
	"Push your bottom teeth forward."	Place two fingers against chin and apply pressure backward.
	"Move your jaw from side to side."	Place one finger on left cheek and apply pressure to right.

*Apply resistance only in the absence of abnormal muscle tone.

Adapted from Alta Bates Hospital Rehabilitation Services: Bedside Dysphagia Evaluation Protocol. Berkeley, Calif, Alta Bates Hospital, 1999; Community Hospital of Los Gatos, Rehabilitation Services: Dysphagia Protocol, Los Gatos, Calif, Community Hospital of Los Gatos, 1999; Logemann J: *Evaluation and treatment of swallowing disorders.* Austin, Tex, Pro-Ed, 1998; and Miller R: Clinical examination for dysphagia. In Groher M: *Dysphagia: Diagnosis and management,* 3rd ed. Newton, Mass, Butterworth-Heinemann, 1997, pp 169-190.

TABLE 3-18   Inner Oral Motor Assessment

Function	Instruction to Client	Testing Procedure*
Tongue		
Protrusion	"Stick out your tongue."	Apply slight resistance toward the back of the throat with tongue blade after client exhibits full range of motion.
Lateralization	"Move your tongue from side to side." "Touch your tongue to your inside cheek—right, then left; move your tongue up and down."	Apply slight resistance in opposite direction of motion with tongue blade. Using finger on outside of cheek, push against tongue inwardly.
Tipping	"Touch your tongue to your upper lip." "Open your mouth. Touch your tongue behind your front teeth."	With tongue blade between tongue tip and lip, apply downward pressure. With tongue blade between tongue and teeth, apply downward pressure on tongue.
Dipping	"Touch your tongue behind your bottom teeth."	With tongue blade between tongue and bottom teeth, apply upward pressure.
Humping	"Say, 'ng'; say, 'ga.'" "Run your tongue along the roof of your mouth, front or back."	Observe for humping of tongue against hard palate. Tongue should flow from front to back. Observe for symmetry and ease of movement.
Swallow		
Hard palate	"Open your mouth and hold it open."	Using flashlight, gently examine for sensitivity by walking finger from front to back.
Soft palate	"Say, 'ah' for as long as you can (5 seconds)." "Change pitch up an octave."	Observe for tightening of faucial arches, elevation of uvula. Using laryngeal mirror, stroke juncture of hard and soft palate to elicit palatal reflex. Observe for upward and backward movement of soft palate.
Hyoid elevation	"Can you swallow for me?"	Place finger at base of client's tongue underneath the chin, and feel for (base of tongue) elevation just before movement of the larynx.
Laryngeal		
Range of motion	"I am going to move your Adam's apple side to side."	Grasp larynx by placing fingers and thumb along sides. Move larynx gently side to side; evaluate for ease and symmetry of movement.
Elevation	"Can you swallow for me?"	Place fingers along the larynx: first finger at hyoid, second finger at top of larynx, and so on. Feel for quick and smooth elevation of larynx as the client swallows.

Continued

TABLE 3-18 Inner Oral Motor Assessment—cont'd

Function	Instruction to Client	Testing Procedure*
Cough		
Voluntary	"Can you cough?"	Observe for ease and strength of movement, loudness of cough, swallow after cough.
Reflexive	"Take a deep breath."	As client holds breath, using palm of hand, push downward (toward stomach) on the sternum. Evaluate strength of reaction.

*Apply resistance in absence of abnormal muscle tone.

Adapted from Community Hospital of Los Gatos, Rehabilitation Services: Dysphagia Protocol. Los Gatos, Calif, Community Hospital of Los Gatos, 1999; Coombes K: Swallowing dysfunction in hemiplegia and head injury. Course presented by International Clinical Educators, Aug 24-27, 1986, and Aug 24-28, 1987, Los Gatos, Calif; Hislop H, Montgomery J, Connelly B: *Daniels and worthington's muscle testing: Techniques of manual examination*, 6th ed. Philadelphia, WB Saunders, 1995; Miller R: Clinical examination for dysphagia. In Groher M: *Dysphagia: Diagnosis and management*, 3rd ed. Newton, Mass, Butterworth-Heinemann, 1997, pp 169-190; Schulze-Delrieu K, Miller R: Clinical assessment of dysphagia. In Perlman A, Schulze-Delrieu K (eds): Deglutition and *its disorders: Anatomy, physiology, clinical diagnosis and management*. San Diego, Calif, Singular, 1997, pp 125-152.

Clinical Assessment of Swallowing

1. Is the client alert and able to participate in a swallowing assessment?
2. Does the client maintain adequate trunk and head control, with or without assistance?
3. Does the client display adequate tongue control to form a cohesive bolus and move the bolus through the oral cavity?
4. Is the larynx mobile enough to elevate quickly and with sufficient force during the swallow?
5. Can the client handle the saliva with minimal drooling?
6. Does the client have a productive cough, strong enough to expel any material that may enter the airway?

If the answer is "yes" to all these questions, the therapist may assess the client's oral and swallow control with a variety of food consistencies.

INDICATORS OF EATING AND SWALLOWING DYSFUNCTION

1. Difficulty with bringing food to the mouth
2. Difficulty or inability to shape food into a cohesive bolus with prolonged chewing
   - Loss of food or liquids from the mouth, drooling
   - Loss of food or liquids from the nose (nasal regurgitation)

3. Coughing or frequent throat clearing before, during, or after the swallow
4. Wet or gurgling voice quality after eating or drinking
5. Changes in mealtime behaviors
   - Food residue remaining in the mouth (cheeks, gums, teeth, tongue)
   - Loss of appetite, dehydration or weight loss
   - Discomfort or pain when swallowing
   - Difficulty breathing while eating
   - Unusual head or neck movements when swallowing
6. Delayed or absent swallow response
7. Weak cough
8. Reflux of food after meals
   - Heartburn
   - Changes in eating—for example, eating slowly or avoiding social occasions
   - Food avoidance
   - Prolonged meal times
   - Recurrent episodes of pneumonia

The presence of any swallowing dysfunction can lead to aspiration pneumonia. The following are acute symptoms of aspiration occurring immediately after the swallow:

- Any change in the client's color, particularly if the airway is obstructed
- Prolonged coughing
- Gurgling voice and extreme breathiness or loss of voice

During the 24 hours immediately after the swallow, the therapist and medical staff must observe the client for additional signs of aspiration. These may include a nasal drip, increase in profuse drooling of a clear liquid, and temperature of 100°F or higher, which may not have been evident during the clinical examination. If aspiration pneumonia develops, the client must be reevaluated for a change in diet levels or taken off the feeding program, if necessary. An alternative feeding method may be necessary to ensure adequate hydration and nutrition.

TABLE 3-19 Dysphagia, Level 1: Dysphagia Pureed

Food Group	Recommended	Avoid
Cereals and breads	Pureed bread mixes, pregelled slurried breads, pancakes, or French toast Smooth, homogenous cooked cereals, creamed wheat or rice, Malto Meal. Cereals should have a pudding-like consistency	All other breads, rolls, crackers, muffins, All dry cereals and any cereals with lumps Oatmeal
Eggs	Custard, puréed eggs	All others
Fruits	Puréed fruits or well-mashed bananas Applesauce	All others; any whole fruits (fresh, frozen, canned)
Potatoes and starches	Mashed potatoes with gravy, puréed potatoes with gravy, butter, margarine, or sour cream Pureed well-cooked noodles, pasta or rice; must be puréed to a smooth, homogenous consistency	All others
Soups	Soups that have been puréed in a blender or strained. May need to be thickened. Thickened, strained cream soups (to a consistency of puréed vegetables)	Soups that have chunks or lumps
Vegetables	Puréed vegetables without lumps, chunks, pulp, or seeds	All vegetables that have not been puréed
Meat and meat substitutes	Puréed meat Puréed poultry with gravy Softened tofu mixed with moisture Hummus or other puréed legume spread	Whole or ground meats, fish, or poultry Cottage cheese, cheese Peanut butter, unless puréed into foods
Desserts	Smooth puddings, custards, yogurt, puréed desserts and soufflés	Ices, gelatins, frozen juice bars, bread and rice pudding, yogurt with fruit All other desserts **These foods are considered thin liquids and should be avoided if thin liquids are restricted.** Frozen malts, milk shakes, frozen yogurt, ice cream, sherbet, gelatin
Fats	Butter, margarine, strained gravy, sour cream, mayonnaise, cream cheese, whipped topping	All fats with chunky additives

Adapted from American Dietetic Association: National Dysphagia Diet: Standardization for Optimal Care. Chicago, American Dietetic Association, 2002; American Occupational Therapy Association: AOTA Resource Guide: Feeding and Dysphagia. Rockville, Md, American Occupational Therapy Association, 1997; Avery-Smith W: An occupational therapist coordinated dysphagia program. Occup Ther Pract 3:10, 1998; Community Hospital of Los Gatos, Rehabilitation Services: Dysphagia Protocol. Los Gatos, Calif, Community Hospital of Los Gatos, 2003; Curran J: Nutritional considerations in dysphagia. In Groher M (ed): Dysphagia: Diagnosis and management, 3rd ed. Newton, Mass, Butterworth-Heinemann, 1997, pp 289-312; and Rader T, Rende B: Swallowing disorders: What families should know. Tucson, Ariz, Communication Skill Builders, 1993.

TABLE 3-20 Dysphagia, Level 2: Dysphagia Mechanically Altered Characteristics (Mechanical Soft)

Food Group	Recommended	Avoid
Cereals and breads	Cooked refined cereals with little texture (e.g., oatmeal) Slightly moistened dry cereals with little texture (e.g., Corn Flakes, Rice Krispies) Soft pancakes with syrup French toast without crust Graham crackers	Very coarse cooked cereals that may contain seeds or nuts Whole-grain dry or coarse cereals All others
Eggs	Poached, scrambled, or soft eggs (egg yolks should be moist and mashable with butter, not runny) Souffles—may have small chunks	Hard cooked or fried eggs
Fruits	Soft canned or cooked fruits without seeds or skill Soft, ripe bananas Baked apple (no skin)	Fruits with seeds, coarse skins, fibers; fruits with pits, raisins, grapes, all raw fruits except those listed
Potatoes and starches	Well-cooked, moistened, boiled, baked, or mashed potatoes Well-cooked noodles in sauce	Potato skins and chips, fried potatoes, rice
Soups	Soups with easy to chew or easy to swallow soft meats or vegetables (particle size < $^1/_2$ inch) Cream soups	Soups that have large chunks of meat or vegetables Soups with rice, corn, peas
Vegetables	Soft, well-cooked vegetables; should be easily mashed with a fork	All raw vegetables Cooked corn and pea Broccoli, cabbage, brussels sprouts, asparagus, or other fibrous, nontender cooked vegetables
Meat and meat substitutes	Moistened ground or cooked meat, poultry, or fish May be served with gravy Casseroles without rice Soft, moist lasagna, moist macaroni and cheese Moist meatballs, meat loaf, or fish Tuna or egg salad without large chunks, celery, or onion Cottage cheese, smooth quiche Tofu All meats or protein substitutes should be served with sauces or moistened to help maintain cohesiveness in the oral cavity	Dry, tough meats (e.g., bacon, sausage, hot dogs) Peanut butter Dry casseroles Pizza Sandwiches All other cheeses

Continued

TABLE 3-20 Dysphagia, Level 2: Dysphagia Mechanically Altered Characteristics (Mechanical Soft)—cont'd

Food Group	Recommended	Avoid
Desserts	Pudding and custard Soft fruit pies with bottom crust only Crisps and cobblers without seeds or nuts Canned fruit (excluding pineapple) Soft, moist cakes with icing Pregelled cookies or soft moist cookies "dunked" in milk, coffee, or other liquid	Dry, coarse cakes or cookies Anything with nuts, seeds, coconut, pineapple, or dried fruit Rice or bread pudding
Fats	Butter, margarine, strained gravy, sour cream, mayonnaise, cream cheese, whipped topping	All fats with chunky additives

Adapted from American Dietetic Association: National Dysphagia Diet: Standardization for Optimal Care. Chicago, American Dietetic Association, 2002; American Occupational Therapy Association: AOTA Resource Guide: Feeding and Dysphagia. Rockville, Md, American Occupational Therapy Association, 1997; Avery-Smith W: An occupational therapist coordinated dysphagia program. *Occup Ther Pract* 3:10, 1998; Community Hospital of Los Gatos, Rehabilitation Services: Dysphagia Protocol. Los Gatos, Calif, Community Hospital of Los Gatos, 2003; Curran J: Nutritional considerations in dysphagia. In Groher M (ed): *Dysphagia: Diagnosis and management*, 3rd ed. Newton, Mass, Butterworth-Heinemann, 1997, pp 289-312; and Rader T, Rende B: *Swallowing disorders: What families should know.* Tucson, Ariz, Communication Skill Builders, 1993.

TABLE 3-21 Dysphagia, Level 3: Dysphagia Advanced

Food Group	Recommended	Avoid
Cereals and breads	All well-moistened cereals Any well-moistened breads, muffins, pancakes, waffles Add butter, margarine, syrup, to moisten	Coarse or dry cereals such as shredded wheat Dry toast, crackers Crusty bread such as French bread, hard rolls Popcorn
Eggs	Eggs, prepared any way	
Fruits	All canned and cooked fruit Soft, peeled fresh fruit, without seeds Soft berries	Difficult to chew fresh fruits such as apples or pears Stringy, high-pulp fruits such as papaya or pineapple Uncooked dried fruit Fruit with seeds or coarse skins
Potatoes and starches	All, including rice and fried potatoes	Potato skins Tough, crisp-fried potatoes
Soups	All soups except those on the Avoid list	Soups with tough meats Corn or clam chowders Soups with large chunks (>1 inch)
Vegetables	All cooked, tender vegetables Shredded lettuce	All raw vegetables, except shredded lettuce Cooked corn Nontender, stringy, cooked vegetables
Meat and meat substitutes	Thin-sliced tender or ground meats and poultry Well-moistened fish Casseroles with small chunks of meat, ground meats, or tender meats	Tough, dry meats and poultry
Desserts	All except those on the Avoid list	Dry, coarse cakes or cookies Anything with nuts, seeds, coconut, pineapple, or dried fruit
Fats	All except those on the Avoid list	All fats with chunky additives

Adapted from American Dietetic Association: National Dysphagia Diet: Standardization for Optimal Care. Chicago, American Dietetic Association, 2002; American Occupational Therapy Association: AOTA Resource Guide: Feeding and Dysphagia. Rockville, Md, American Occupational Therapy Association, 1997; Avery-Smith W: An occupational therapist coordinated dysphagia program. Occup Ther Pract 3:10, 1998; Community Hospital of Los Gatos, Rehabilitation Services: Dysphagia Protocol. Los Gatos, Calif, Community Hospital of Los Gatos, 2003; Curran J: Nutritional considerations in dysphagia. In Groher M (ed): Dysphagia: Diagnosis and management, 3rd ed. Newton, Mass, Butterworth-Heinemann, 1997, pp 289-312; and Rader T, Rende B: Swallowing disorders: What families should know. Tucson, Ariz, Communication Skill Builders, 1993.

TABLE 3-22 Liquids

Liquid Consistency	Examples
Thin liquids	Water, ice chips Coffee, tea Milk Hot chocolate Fruit juices Broth or consommé Gelatin dessert Ice cream Sherbet
Nectar-like	Nectars Extra thick milkshake Extra thick eggnog Strained creamed soups Yougurt and milk blended V-8 juice
Honey-like	Nectar thickened with banana Nectar thickened with puréed fruit Regular applesauce with juice Eggnog with baby cereal Creamed soup with mashed potatoes Commercial thickener
Spoon-thick	Commercial thickener

Adapted from American Dietetic Association: National Dysphagia Diet: Standardization for Optimal Care. Chicago, American Dietetic Association, 2002; American Occupational Therapy Association: AOTA Resource Guide: Feeding and Dysphagia. Rockville, Md, American Occupational Therapy Association, 1997; Avery-Smith W: An occupational therapist coordinated dysphagia program. *Occup Ther Pract* 3:10, 1998; Community Hospital of Los Gatos, Rehabilitation Services: Dysphagia Protocol. Los Gatos, Calif, Community Hospital of Los Gatos, 2003; Curran J: Nutritional considerations in dysphagia. In Groher M (ed): *Dysphagia: Diagnosis and management*, 3rd ed. Newton, Mass, Butterworth-Heinemann, 1997, pp 289-312; and Rader T, Rende B: *Swallowing disorders: What families should know.* Tucson, Ariz, Communication Skill Builders, 1993.

TABLE 3-23   Dysphagic Treatment: Oral Preparatory Stage

Structure	Symptoms	Problem	Prefeeding Technique	Feeding Technique
Trunk	Leaning to one side	Decreased trunk tone Ataxia Increased trunk tone Poor body awareness in perceptual space	Facilitate trunk strength Exercises at midline Have client clasp hands, lean down, and touch foot, middle, other foot; rotate trunk with hands clasped and shoulders flexed to decrease or normalize tone	Assist client to hold correct position; assist with head control Assist client to hold correct feeding position; provide with perceptual boundary; consider lateral trunk support
	Hips sliding forward out of chair	Increased tone in hip extensors Poor body awareness in space	See previous entry above Provide firm seating surface	Adjust positioning so that client leans slightly forward at hips, arms forward on table
Head	Inability to hold head in midline	Decreased tone Weakness	Facilitate strength through neck and head exercises in flexion, extension, and lateral flexion	Assist with head control
	Inability to move head	Increased tone Poor range of motion	Tone reduction of head, shoulders, and trunk Facilitate normal movement Myofascial release techniques Soft tissue mobilization	Assist with head control
Upper extremity	Spillage of food from utensils	Decreased tone Apraxia Decreased coordination	Facilitate increased tone through correct weight bearing, sweeping, or tapping muscle belly of desired muscle	Guide client through correct movement pattern Provide adaptive equipment or utensils as needed
	Inability to self-feed	Increased tone Abnormal movement patterns Weakness or decreased motor control	Reduce proximal tone with scapula mobilization, weight bearing through arm Strengthening exercises Facilitation of normal movement	Guide client through correct movement pattern Provide adaptive equipment or utensils as needed

Continued

TABLE 3-23 Dysphagic Treatment: Oral Preparatory Stage—cont'd

Structure	Symptoms	Problem	Prefeeding Technique	Feeding Technique
Face head	Drooling, food spill-age from mouth	Decreased lip control Poor lip closure secondary to decreased tone, poor sensation Apraxia	Place a wet tongue blade between client's lips; ask client to hold tongue blade while therapist tries to pull it out Vibrate lips with back of electric toothbrush down cheek and across lips Lip exercises: movements described in outer oral motor evaluation; client performs repetitions 2-3 times daily Blow bubbles into glass of liquid with straw	Using side handgrip for head control, the therapist approximates lip closure by guiding and assisting with jaw closure Have client use a straw when drinking liquids until control improves Place food to unimpaired side Use cold food or liquids
		Decreased sensation	Fan lips so that client feels drool or wetness on lips or chin to increase awareness	Teach client to pat mouth (versus wiping mouth) and chin every few bites or sips
Tongue	Pocketing of food in cheeks or sulci Poor bolus formation	Poor tongue control for lateralization or tipping Decreased tone Poor sensation	Tongue exercises: use movements described in inner oral motor evaluation	Avoid crumbly foods Stroke client's outside cheek where pocketing occurs, with index finger back and up toward client's ear; instruct client to check cheek for pocketing
	Retracted tongue	Increased tone Retracted jaw	Tongue range of motion: wrap tip of tongue in wet gauze; gently pull tongue forward, side to side and up and down; move slowly Pull tongue wrapped in wet gauze forward past front teeth, using index and middle fingers to vibrate tongue back and forth sideways to decrease tone and facilitate protrusion	Avoid crumbly foods Reduce tone as needed during meal Double swallow Resist head extension to facilitate jaw opening Resist head flexion to facilitate jaw closure

Adapted from American Occupational Therapy Association: Am J Occup Ther, 1996; Avery-Smith W: Management of neurologic disorders: the first feeding session. In Groher M, editor: *Dysphagia: Diagnosis and management*, ed 3, Newton, Mass, 1997, Butterworth-Heinemann Publishers; Bobath B: *Adult hemiplegia: Evaluation and treatment*, ed 2, London, 1978, William Heinemann Medical Books; Community Hospital of Los Gatos, Rehabilitation Services: Dysphagia protocol, Los Gatos, Calif, 2003; Coombes K: Swallowing dysfunction in hemiplegia and head injury. Course presented by International Clinical Educators, Aug 24-27, 1986, and Aug 24-28, 1987, Los Gatos, Calif; Davies P: *Steps to follow*. New York, Springer-Verlag, 1985; Farber S: *Neurorehabilitation: A multisensory approach*, Philadelphia, 1982, WB Saunders; Logemann J: *Manual for the videofluorographic study of swallowing*, ed 2, Austin, Tex, 1993, Pro-Ed.

TABLE 3-24 Dysphagic Treatment: Oral Stage

Structure	Symptoms	Problem	Prefeeding Technique	Feeding Technique
Tongue	Slow oral transit Tongue retraction	Poor anterior to posterior movement; decreased tone, poor sensation Increased tone	Practice "ng·ga" sounds Grasping tongue wrapped in gauze, pull it forward past front teeth; use finger or tongue blade to vibrate base of tongue back and forth sideways Improve tongue range of motion	Tuck chin toward chest Position food in center, midtongue Avoid crumbly foods Use cold or hot foods instead of warm Correct positioning Place index finger at base of tongue under chin; stroke up and forward
	Slow oral transit time Inability to channel food back toward pharynx	Inability to form central groove in tongue Apraxia	Grasping tongue wrapped in gauze, pull forward to front teeth; stroke firmly down middle of tongue with edge of tongue blade	Tuck chin toward chest Position food in center, midtongue Avoid crumbly foods Use cold or hot foods instead of warm Correct positioning Place index finger at base of tongue under chin; stroke up and forward
	Repetitive movement of tongue; food is pushed out front of mouth	Tongue thrust	Facilitate tongue retraction to bring tongue back into normal resting position; vibrate on either side of the frenulum found inside the mouth, under the tongue with finger Increase jaw control; teach isolated tongue movements	Correct positioning Place food away from midline of tongue toward back of mouth Provide downward and forward pressure to back of tongue with spoon after food placement
	Food falls off tongue into sulci or food remains on tongue without client awareness	Poor sensation	Ice tongue with ice chips placed in gauze to prevent ice chips from slipping into pharynx Brush tongue with toothbrush to stimulate receptors	Use foods with high viscosity or density Alternate presentation of cold and hot foods during meal
	Slow oral transit time; food remains on hard palate; coughing before swallow	Poor tongue elevation; decreased tone Decreased sensation Increased tone	Ask client to practice "k," "g," "n," "d," and "t" sounds Lightly touch tongue blade or soft toothbrush to roof of mouth at back of tongue; instruct client to press spot with tongue; resist movement with blade or brush to increase strength Vibrate tongue at base below chin; provide quick stretch by pushing down on base of tongue	Correct positioning With finger under chin at base of tongue, move finger upward and forward to facilitate elevation Avoid crumbly foods Double swallow

Continued

TABLE 3-24 Dysphagic Treatment: Oral Stage—cont'd

Structure	Symptoms	Problem	Prefeeding Technique	Feeding Technique
	Slow oral transit time because client is unable to elevate tongue to push food to hard palate Food remains on back of tongue Coughing before the swallow Retracted tongue	Decreased range of motion Soft tissue shortening	Tone tongue with gauze reduction; grasping wrapped tongue forward with around tip, pull finger or tongue blade Apply pressure to base of tongue right to left Grasping base of tongue under chin between two fingers, move it back and forth to decrease toneTone reduction Range of motion exercises Place a variety of tastes on lips to facilitate tongue-licking lips	Adjust correct positioning by increasing forward flexion at hips, arms forward to decrease tone Reduce tone as needed; give client breaks because tone increases with effort With finger under chin at base of tongue, move finger upward and forward to facilitate tongue elevation

Adapted from Community Hospital of Los Gatos, Rehabilitation Services: Dysphagia Protocol. Los Gatos, Calif, Community Hospital of Los Gatos, 2003; Coombes K: Swallowing dysfunction in hemiplegia and head injury. Course presented by International Clinical Educators, Aug 24-27, 1986, and Aug 24-28, 1987, Los Gatos, Calif; Davies P: *Steps to follow*. New York, Springer-Verlag, 1985; Farber S: *Neurorehabilitation: A multisensory approach*, Philadelphia, WB Saunders, 1982; Logemann J: *Evaluation and treatment of swallowing disorders*, 2nd ed. Austin, Tex, Pro-Ed, 1998; Martin BJW: Treatment of dysphagia in adults. In Cherney L (ed): *Clinical management of dysphagia in adults and children*, 2nd ed. Gaithersburg, Md, Aspen, 1994, pp; Silverman EH, Elfant IL: Am J Occup Ther 1979.

TABLE 3-25 Dysphagia Treatment: Pharyngeal Stage

Structure	Symptoms	Problem	Prefeeding Technique	Feeding Technique
Soft palate	Tight voice; nasal regurgitation Air felt through nose or mist seen on mirror when client says "ah" Decreased tone Nasal speech	Increased tone Decreased tone Rigidity	Facilitate normal head/neck positioning Have client tuck chin into therapist's cupped hand, then push into hand as therapist applies resistance; client says, "ah" afterward; speed and height of uvula elevation should increase; follow by thermal application	Facilitate normal head and neck positioning With head and neck in midline, have client tuck chin slightly to decrease rate of food entering into pharynx
	Delayed swallow	Decreased triggering of swallow response	Thermal application: using a laryngeal mirror #00 after being placed in ice water or chips for 10 seconds, touch base of faucial arch; repeat up to 10 times; process can be repeated several times a day	Alternate presentation of food; start very cold substance, then warm; cold substance can increase sensitivity of faucial arches; tuck chin slightly forward to prevent bolus entering airway
Hyoid	Delayed elevation of hyoid bone Poor tongue elevation Tongue retraction	Delayed swallow Incomplete swallow Abnormal tongue tone; poor range of motion	Increase tongue humping because elevation of tongue and hyoid stimulates triggering of response Tone reduction	Place index finger under chin at base of tongue and push up forward to facilitate tongue elevation
Pharynx	Coughing after swallow	Decreased pharyngeal movement Penetration into laryngeal vestibule	None	If appropriate, alternate presentation of liquid with stage II or stage III solids; liquid material moves solids through pharynx
	Coating of pharynx seen on videofluoroscopy Gurgling voice	Pharyngeal weakness	Isometric or resistive head and neck exercises	Have client take second dry swallow to clear valleculae and pyriform sinuses Tilt head to stronger side Supraglottic swallow
	Seen on videofluoroscopy, anteroposterior view; material residue seen on one side; weak or hoarse voice	Unilateral pharyngeal movement	None	Compensatory technique for clients with low tone: have client turn head toward affected side during swallow to prevent pooling in affected pyriform sinuses; evaluate technique against its effect on client positioning and tone in trunk, upper extremities

Continued

TABLE 3-25 Dysphagia Treatment: Pharyngeal Stage—cont'd

Structure	Symptoms	Problem	Prefeeding Technique	Feeding Technique
Larynx	Coughing, choking after swallow	Decreased laryngeal elevation Decreased tone Weakness	Quickly ice up sides of larynx; ask client to swallow; assist movement by guiding larynx upward Vibrate laryngeal musculature from under chin, downward on each side to sternal notch	Teach client to clear throat immediately after swallow to move residual Use supraglottic swallow, Mendelsohn maneuver, effortful swallow
	Noisy or audible swallow	Increased tone Rigidity Uncoordinated swallow	Range of motion—place fingers and thumb along both sides of larynx and gently move it back and forth until movement is smooth and easy/tone decreased Using chipped ice, form pack in washcloth and place around larynx for 5 min	Placing fingers and thumb along both sides of larynx, assist client with upward elevation before swallow Double swallow
Trachea	Continuous coughing before, during, after swallow	Aspiration—before: poor tongue control; during: delayed swallow response; after: decreased pharyngeal movement	Teach client how to produce a voluntary cough; ask client to take a deep breath and cough while breathing out; therapist uses palm of hand to push downward (toward stomach) on the sternum	Encourage client to keep coughing; facilitate reflexive cough; push downward on sternum as client breathes out; suction client if problem increases Push into client's sternal notch to assist with cough
	Client grabs or reaches for throat Reddening in the face No voice or cough	Blocked airway	None	Perform Heimlich maneuver Seek medical assistance

Adapted from Community Hospital of Los Gatos, Rehabilitation Services: Dysphagia Protocol. Los Gatos, Calif, Community Hospital of Los Gatos, 1999; Coombes K: Swallowing dysfunction in hemiplegia and head injury. Course presented by International Clinical Educators, Aug 24-27, 1986, and Aug 24-28, 1987, Los Gatos, Calif; Davies P: *Steps to follow.* New York, Springer-Verlag, 1985; Katzke-McDonald M, Post E, Davis P: *Dysphagia,* 1996; Logemann J: *Evaluation and treatment of swallowing disorders,* 2nd ed. Austin, Tex, Pro-Ed, 1998; Martin BJW: Treatment of dysphagia in adults. In Cherney L (ed): *Clinical management of dysphagia in adults and children,* 2nd ed. Gaithersburg, Md, Aspen, 1994, *pp* ; Schulze-Delrieu K, Miller R: Clinical assessment of dysphagia. In Perlman A, Schulze-Delrieu K (eds): *Deglutition and its disorders: Anatomy, physiology, clinical diagnosis and management.* San Diego, Calif, Singular, 1997, pp 125-152; and Smith C, Logemann J, Colangelo L, et al: Incidence and patient characteristics associated with silent aspiration in the acute care setting. *Dysphagia* 14:1-7, 1999.

TABLE 3-26 Dysphagia Treatment: Esophageal Stage

Structure	Symptoms	Problem	Prefeeding Technique	Feeding Technique
Esophagus	Frequent regurgitation of food or liquid and coughing or choking after the swallow: material collecting in a side pocket in esophagus	Esophageal diverticulum	Requires a medical diagnosis; problem can be seen through traditional barium x-ray examination Surgical correction is needed	Report symptoms to medical staff (therapist cannot treat)
	Regurgitation of food, coughing, or choking on food after the swallow: inability of food to pass through the pharynx, esophagus, or stomach	Partial or total obstruction of the pharynx or esophagus Impaired esophageal peristalsis	Requires a medical diagnosis; problem can be seen through traditional barium x-ray examination Surgical correction is needed	Report symptoms to medical staff (therapist cannot treat)

Adapted from Coombes K: Swallowing dysfunction in hemiplegia and head injury. Course presented by International Clinical Educators, Aug 24-27, 1986, and Aug 24-28, 1987, Los Gatos, Calif; Davies P: *Steps to follow.* New York, Springer-Verlag, 1985; Logemann J: *Evaluation and treatment of swallowing disorders.* Austin, Tex, Pro-Ed, 1998; Smith C, Logemann J, Colangelo L, et al: *Dysphagia,* 1999; Martin B: Treatment of dysphagia in adults. In Cherney L, editor: *Clinical management of dysphagia in adults and children,* Gaithersburg, Md, 1994, Aspen. Workman J, Pillsbury H, Hulka G: Surgical interventions in dysphagia. In Groher M: *Dysphagia: diagnosis and management,* ed 3, Newton, Mass, 1977, Butterworth-Heinemann.

TABLE 3-27 Bolus Textures and Swallow Problems

Texture	Disorders for Which This Texture is Most Appropriate
Thin liquid	Tongue dysfunction (ROM, strength, coordination) Reduced tongue base retraction Reduced pharyngeal wall contraction Reduced laryngeal elevation Reduced cricopharyngeal opening
Thickened liquid	Tongue dysfunction (ROM, strength, coordination) Delayed pharyngeal swallow
Pureed	Oral motor impairment Delayed pharyngeal swallow Impaired cognition Decreased endurance
Mechanical soft	Oral motor impairment (decreased chew) Decreased endurance

Adapted from Logemann J: *Evaluation and treatment of swallowing disorders.* Austin, Tex, Pro-Ed, 1998.

The Occupational Therapy Process: Implementation of Interventions

Pain Management

Acute pain and its associated physiologic, psychological, and behavioral responses are typically caused by tissue irritation or damage in relation to injury, disease, disability, or medical or rehabilitative procedures. It has a well-defined pain onset. Acute pain serves a biologic purpose, directing attention to injury, irritation, or disease and signaling the need for immobilization and protection of a body part. Fortunately, acute pain is predictable and usually responds to medication and treatment of the underlying cause of pain.

Chronic or persistent pain may begin as acute pain or may be more insidious and endure beyond the point at which an underlying pathologic condition can be identified. Increased sympathetic nervous system activity does not continue. Chronic pain does not appear to serve a biologic purpose. It is unpredictable and not amenable to routine interventions. Chronic pain often produces significant changes in personality, lifestyle, and functional ability.

BOX 4-1   Examples of Pain Intensity Scales

Simple Descriptive Pain Intensity Scale*
No pain
Mild pain
Moderate pain
Severe pain
Very severe pain
Worst pain possible

Numerical Pain Intensity Scale, 0-10*
This ranges from no pain (rated as 0) to moderate pain (2-9) to worst pain possible (10).

Visual Analogue Scale (VAS)†
This ranges from "no pain" to "pain as bad as it could possibly be."

---

*If used as a graphic rating scale, a 10-cm baseline is recommended.
†A 10-cm baseline is recommended for VAS scales.
Adapted from U.S. Department of Health and Human Services, Acute Pain Management Guideline Panel: *Acute pain management in adults: Operative procedures. Quick reference guide for clinicians* (AHCPR Publ. No. 92-0019). Rockville, Md, U.S. Government Printing Office, 1995.

BOX 4-2 Pain Interference Scales

These numerical pain intensity scales range from 0-10.

A. *In the past week,* how much has pain interfered with your daily activities?

0	1	2	3	4	5	6	7	8	9	10

No
interference

Unable to carry out
any activities

B. *In the past week,* how much has pain interfered with your ability to take part in recreational, social, and family activities?

0	1	2	3	4	5	6	7	8	9	10

No
interference

Unable to carry out
any activities

C. *In the past week,* how much has pain interfered with your ability to work (including housework)?

0	1	2	3	4	5	6	7	8	9	10

No
interference

Unable to carry out
any activities

From National Institutes of Health, National Institute of Child Health and Human Development, National Institute of Neurological Disorders and Stroke: Ongoing Research; Management of Chronic Pain in Rehabilitation (Grant No. 1, PO1 HD/NS33988).

BOX 4-3 Glossary

Nociception: The detection of potentially tissue-damaging thermal or mechanical energy by specialized nerve endings.

Pain: An unpleasant sensory and emotional experience associated with actual or potential tissue damage.

Pain Behavior: Observable and measurable behaviors used by the client to communicate the experience of pain to others.

Suffering: An unwanted condition and the corresponding negative emotion

---

Therapeutic Occupations and Modalities

Purposeful Occupation and Activity

When an intervention plan is being developed, the inherent goals of the activity, client's level of interest in the activity, and meaning of the activity and its product are important considerations in the ultimate effectiveness of the media and methods selected for intervention. Purposeful activities are used, or adapted for use, to meet one or more of the following therapeutic objectives: (1) to develop or maintain strength, endurance, work tolerance, range of motion (ROM), and coordination; (2) to practice and use voluntary automatic movement in goal-directed tasks; (3) to provide for purposeful use of and general exercise to affected parts; (4) to explore vocational potential or train in work skills; (5) to improve sensation, perception, and cognition; (6) to improve socialization skills and enhance emotional growth and development; and (7) to increase independence in occupational role performance.

GRADING OF ACTIVITY

Activities may be graded in many ways to suit the client's needs and meet the intervention objectives. Activities can be graded for increasing strength, range of motion (ROM), endurance and tolerance, coordination, and perceptual, cognitive, and social skills.

- Strength may be graded by an increase or decrease in resistance. Methods include changing the plane of movement from gravity eliminated to against gravity, by adding weights to the equipment or to the client, using tools of increasing weights, grading the texture of the materials from soft to hard or fine to rough, or changing to another more or less resistive activity.
- Activities for increasing or maintaining joint ROM may be graded by positioning materials and equipment to demand greater reach or excursion of joints or by adapting equipment with lengthened handles to facilitate active stretching.
- Endurance may be graded by moving from light to heavy work and increasing the duration of the work period. Standing and walking tolerance may be graded by an increase in the time spent standing to work and an increase in the time and distance spent in activities requiring walking.
- Coordination and muscle control may be graded by decreasing the gross resistive movements and increasing the fine controlled movements required. Dexterity and speed of movement may be graded by practicing at increasing speeds once movement patterns have been mastered.
- In grading cognitive skills, the therapist can begin the treatment program with simple one- or two-step activities that require little judgment, decision making, or problem solving, and progress to activities with several steps that require some judgment or problem-solving processes.
- For grading social interaction, the intervention plan may begin with an activity that demands interaction only with the therapist. The client can progress to activities that require dyadic interaction with another client and, ultimately, to small group activities.

Orthotics

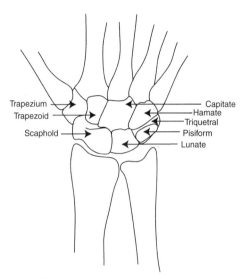

FIGURE 4-1 Skeletal structures of the wrist, dorsal view.

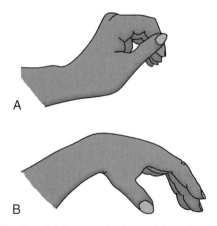

FIGURE 4-2 Tenodesis. **A,** Active wrist extension results in passive finger flexion. **B,** Active wrist flexion results in passive finger extension.

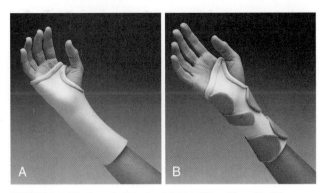

FIGURE 4-3 A, Trim lines of splint extend distal to MP creases and limit finger flexion. **B,** Splint's distal trim lines fall proximal to MP creases (following the oblique angle of the metacarpal heads) and permit full finger flexion.

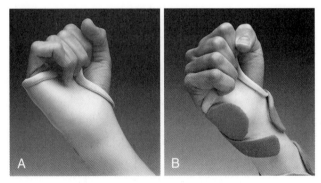

FIGURE 4-4 A, Fourth and fifth digits are prevented from full flexion. **B,** Full finger flexion is possible with proper trim lines.

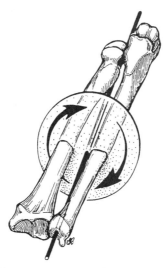

FIGURE 4-5 Axis of motion for supination and pronation extends the length of the forearm. It is centered through the radial head and capitulum and the distal ulnar styloid. (From Colello-Abraham K: *Rehabilitation of the hand,* 3rd ed. St. Louis, Mosby, 1990.)

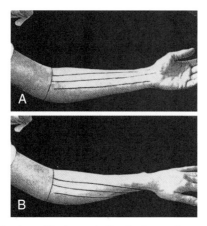

FIGURE 4-6 The shape of the forearm is altered as it moves from supination to pronation. Forearm-based splints must be repositioned to accommodate this if the forearm is rotated during the fabrication process. (From Wilton JC: *Hand splinting: Principles of design and fabrication.* Philadelphia, WB Saunders, 1997.)

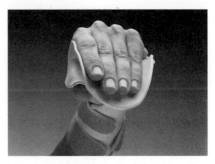

FIGURE 4-7 Oblique angle of transverse arch at MP joints must be accommodated to ensure maintenance of more mobile fourth and fifth digits.

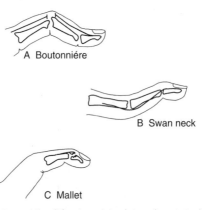

FIGURE 4-8 A, Boutonnière deformity, or joint change characterized by PIP joint flexion and DIP hyperextension. **B,** Swan-neck deformity, or joint change, with PIP hyperextension and DIP joint flexion. **C,** Mallet finger with DIP joint flexion and loss of active extension.

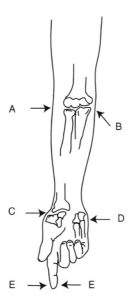

FIGURE 4-9 Potential sites for nerve compression from improperly fitted splints. **A,** Radial nerve. **B,** Ulnar nerve. **C,** Radial digital nerve in anatomical snuffbox. **D,** Ulnar nerve in Guyon's canal. **E,** Digital nerves.

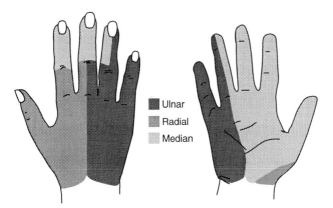

FIGURE 4-10 Sensory distribution in hand. Median nerve distribution includes most of the prehensile surface of the palm.

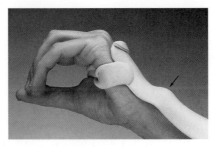

FIGURE 4-11 Relief "bubbled" over the ulnar styloid accomplished by molding plastic over a pad placed on the styloid.

Prehension and Grasp Patterns

LATERAL PREHENSION

In lateral prehension, the pad of the thumb is positioned to contact the radial side of the middle or distal phalanx of the index finger (Fig. 4-12A). Usually, this pattern of prehension is used in holding a pen or eating utensil and holding and turning a key. The short or long opponens splint is used to stabilize the thumb to achieve this prehension pattern.

PALMAR PREHENSION

Palmar prehension is also called a three-jaw chuck pinch. The thumb is positioned in opposition to the index and long fingers (see Fig. 4-12B). The important component of motion in this pattern is thumb rotation, which allows for pad to pad opposition. This prehension pattern is used for lifting objects from a flat surface, holding small objects, and tying a shoe or bow. The short and long opponens splints may also be fabricated to position the thumb in palmar prehension.

TIP PREHENSION

In tip prehension, the interphalangeal (IP) joint of the thumb and the distal interphalangeal (DIP) and proximal interphalangeal (PIP) joints of the finger are flexed to facilitate tip to tip prehension (see Fig. 4-12C). These motions are necessary to pick up a pin or a

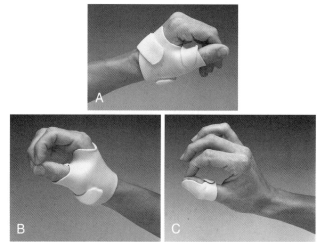

FIGURE 4-12 A, Lateral prehension or key pinch in short opponens splint that positions thumb in lateral opposition to index finger. **B,** Palmar prehension or three-jaw chuck pinch in short opponens that positions thumb in opposition to index and long fingers. **C,** Tip prehension with thumb and index finger in IP blocker that secures the IP joint in slight flexion to assist tip prehension.

coin. It is difficult to substitute for tip prehension because it is rarely a static holding posture. Once a pin is in the hand, tip prehension will convert to palmar prehension to provide more skin surface area to retain a small object. A thumb IP hyperextension block is useful to limit IP hyperextension and to facilitate the IP flexion required for tip prehension.

CYLINDRICAL GRASP

Cylindrical grasp, the most common static grasp pattern, is used to stabilize objects against the palm and the fingers, with the thumb acting as an opposing force (Fig. 4-13A). This pattern is assumed for grasping a hammer, pot handle, drinking glass, or the handhold on a walker or crutch. Static splinting offers little to restore this grasp directly, although positioning the wrist in extension offers greater stability to the hand as it assumes this grasp pattern. However, a dynamic outrigger component can be added to a volar splint to gain increased metacarpophalangeal

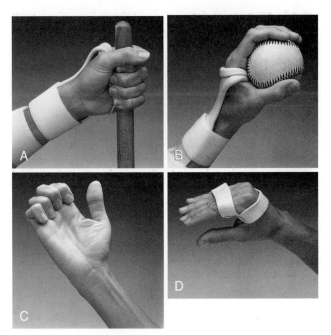

FIGURE 4-13 A, Cylindrical grasp in dorsal splint that stabilizes wrist to increase grip force and minimizes palm covering. **B,** Spherical grasp in dorsal splint. Splint stabilizes wrist to increase grip force and permits metacarpal mobility required for spherical grasp. **C,** Hook grasp does not involve thumb. The grasp pattern is seen in median and ulnar neuropathy; splinting is aimed at correcting rather than augmenting grasp. **D,** Figure-eight splint substitutes for loss of intrinsic function with median and ulnar neuropathy.

(MP) and PIP flexion gently to increase cylindrical grasping ability.

SPHERICAL GRASP

Also called ball grasp, this pattern is assumed for holding a round object, such as a ball or apple. It differs from cylindrical grasp primarily in the positioning of the fourth and fifth digits. In cylindrical grasp, the two ulnar metacarpals are held in greater flexion. In spherical grasp, the two ulnar digits are supported in greater extension to allow a more open hand posture (see Fig. 4-13B). In splinting, to facilitate or support this pattern of grasp, the wrist-stabilizing splint must be trimmed proximal to the distal palmar crease and contoured to allow for the obliquity at the fourth and fifth metacarpal heads.

HOOK GRASP

Hook grasp is the only prehension pattern that does not include the thumb to supply opposition. The MPs are held in extension and the DIP and PIP joints are held in flexion (see Fig. 4-13C). This is the attitude that the hand assumes when holding the handle of a shopping bag, pail, or briefcase. In the nerve-injured hand, splinting is more commonly directed at correcting this posture by flexing the MPs rather than at facilitating it.

INTRINSIC PLUS GRASP

Intrinsic plus grasp is characterized by the positioning of all the MPs of the fingers in flexion, the DIP and PIP joints in full extension, and the thumb in opposition to the third and fourth fingers (see Fig. 4-13D). This pattern is used for grasping and holding large flat objects such as books or plates. Intrinsic plus grasp is often lost in the presence of median or ulnar nerve dysfunction, and a figure-eight or dynamic MP flexion splint is used for substitution (Figs. 4-14 to 4-24).

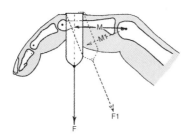

FIGURE 4-14 Tension (F) on the phalanx has a moment arm (M) acting on the joint. Tension (F1) has a smaller moment arm (M1), with less resulting torque, when the angle of approach is not 90 degrees. (From Brand PW, Hollister A: *Clinical mechanics of the hand,* 2nd ed. St. Louis, Mosby, 1993.)

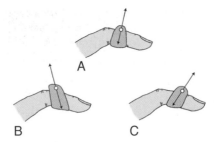

FIGURE 4-15 A, Angle of approach is 90 degrees to middle phalanx, ensuring that the force pulling the PIP joint into extension is not causing distraction or compression. **B,** Angle of approach less than 90 degrees to middle phalanx causes joint compression. **C,** Angle of approach greater than 90 degrees distracts joint.

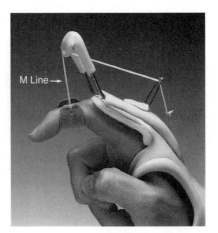

FIGURE 4-16 As dynamic traction acts on ROM at the PIP joint, the splint must be adjusted to maintain 90-degree angle of approach.

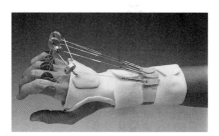

FIGURE 4-17 Forearm-based four-digit outrigger with dynamic extension assist supplied by springs.

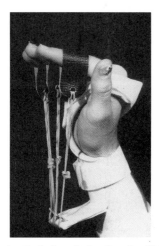

FIGURE 4-18 Dynamic splint for finger flexion. (From Fess EE, Gettle KS, Philips CA, et al: *Hand and upper extremity splinting: Principles and methods,* 3rd ed. St. Louis, Mosby, 2005.)

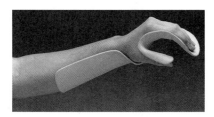

FIGURE 4-19 Single-surface static resting splint positions hand in 20- to 30-degree wrist extension, 45- to 60-degree MP flexion, and 15- to 30-degree PIP and DIP flexion.

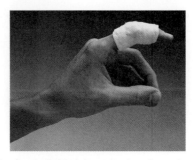

FIGURE 4-20 A series of cylindrical plaster casts is made to reduce flexion contracture at proximal interphalangeal joint.

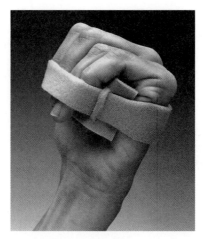

FIGURE 4-21 Static progressive web strap adjusts with hook closure. The patient is taught to adjust the strap as tolerance permits.

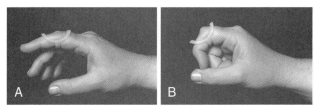

FIGURE 4-22 Oval-eight ring splints. **A,** Ring splint restricts PIP joint hyperextension. **B,** Ring splint allows full flexion.

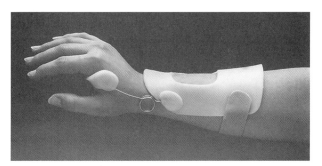

FIGURE 4-23 Spring coil splint substitutes for absent wrist extension in radial nerve injury.

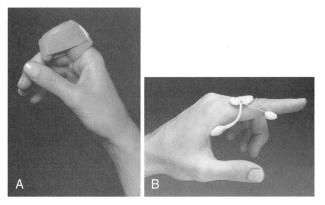

FIGURE 4-24 A, Final flexion strap designed to restore full IP joint flexion provides equal force on all surfaces of the digit. **B,** Three-point pressure splint with spring wire reduces PIP joint flexion contractures of 35 degrees or less.

Indications for Single-Surface Splinting

Single-surface splinting is effective for supporting joints surrounded by weak or flaccid muscles—for example, following a cerebrovascular accident (CVA) or peripheral nerve injury. Because little or no active motion is available, the extra control given by circumferential splinting is not needed, and putting on and taking off the splint will be easier. A single-surface splint is also effective as the base for attaching outriggers in dynamic splinting and for postoperative splints in which the fabrication of a circumferential splint may damage repaired structures (Figs. 4-25 to 4-29).

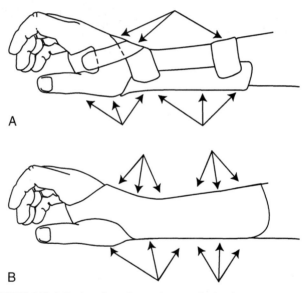

FIGURE 4-25 A, Single-surface splint requires properly placed straps to create three-point pressure systems to secure splint and ensure distribution of pressure. **B,** Circumferential splints create multiple three-point pressure systems to secure splint for immobilization.

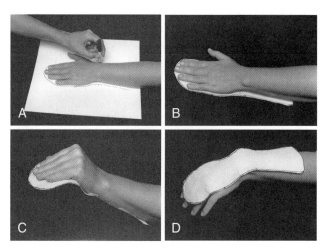

FIGURE 4-26 A, Tracing with pencil perpendicular to arm creates a true size pattern. **B,** Pattern is full length with hand flat. **C,** Pattern is too long when fit onto the volar surface with hand in resting position. **D,** Pattern is too short when fit on dorsum of hand with wrist and fingers in flexion.

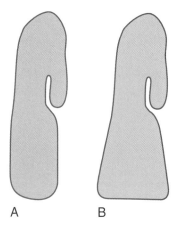

FIGURE 4-27 A, Narrowing the proximal pattern will cause trim lines to drop below midline. **B,** Flaring the proximal border of the splint maintains trim lines at midline.

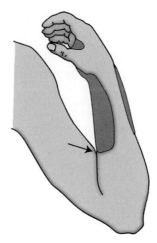

FIGURE 4-28 Length of forearm-based splint is checked by flexing elbow and noting where biceps meets forearm. Splint is trimmed ¼ to ½ inch distal to point of contact.

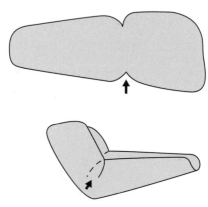

FIGURE 4-29 Drawing darts in elbow pattern allows material to be overlapped and contoured without excess material.

RESISTANCE TO STRETCH

Resistance to stretch describes the extent to which a material resists pulling or stretching. The greater the resistance, the greater the degree of control that the splint maker will have over the material. Materials that resist stretch tend to hold their shape and thickness while warm and can be handled more aggressively without thinning. The more resistive materials are recommended for large splints and for splints made for those who are unable to cooperate in the fabrication process. In contrast, the less resistance to stretch a material has, the more the material is likely to thin during the fabrication process and the more delicately it must be handled. The advantage of stretch is seen in the greater degree of conformability obtained with less effort on the splint maker's part.

CONFORMABILITY OR DRAPE

Resistance to stretch and conformability or drape describe almost the same characteristic—that is, if a material stretches easily, it will have better drape and conformability. The great advantage of materials with a high degree of drape or conformability is that with a light controlled touch or simply the pull of gravity, they readily conform around a part for a precise fit. The disadvantage of materials with a high degree of drape (and generally also low resistance to stretch) is that they tolerate only minimal handling, and care must be taken to prevent overstretching and fingerprints in the material. Materials with a high degree of drape are not recommended for large splints or for uncooperative clients. They are ideal, however, for splinting postoperative clients when minimal pressure is desired and for dynamic splint bases in which conformability secures the splint against migration (movement distally) when components are attached. Materials with a low degree of drape must be handled continuously until the materials are fully cooled to achieve a contoured fit and often will not conform intimately around small parts, such as fingers.

MEMORY

Memory is the ability of a material, when reheated, to return to its original flat shape after it has been stretched and molded. The advantage of high memory in a material is that the splint can be remolded repeatedly without the material thinning and losing strength. Materials with memory require handling throughout the splint-making process because until they are fully cooled and molded, they tend to return to a flat shape. This and the slightly longer cooling time of materials with high memory can be used to advantage with clients who require more aggressive handling to achieve the desired position. Disadvantages of materials with excellent memory are their tendency to return to a flat sheet state when an area is spot-heated for adjustment and their need for longer handling to ensure that they maintain their molded shape until fully cooled.

RIGIDITY VERSUS FLEXIBILITY

Generally, the thicker a thermoplastic and the more plastic its formula contains, the more rigid the material will be. Thermoplastics come in thicknesses from ⅛ inch (3.2 mm) to as thin as ¹⁄₁₆ inch (1.6 mm). The thinner materials and the thermoplastics that contain rubber-like polymers in their formula tend to have greater flexibility in their molded state. Flexibility in a material makes it easier to put on and take off splints and may be desirable for clients unable to tolerate the more unforgiving rigid materials.

BONDING

Bonding is the ability of a material to adhere to itself when warmed and pressed together. Many materials are coated to resist accidental bonding and require solvents or surface scraping to remove the coating to bond. Uncoated materials, which require no solvents or scraping, have very strong bonding properties when two warm pieces are pressed together. Self-bonding is helpful when outriggers or overlapping corners are applied to form acute angles but can be a problem if two pieces adhere accidentally.

SELF-SEALING EDGES

Self-sealing edges are edges that round and seal themselves when heated material is cut. This characteristic produces smooth edges that require no additional finishing, which adds time to the fabrication process. Materials with little or no memory and high conformability generally produce smooth sealed edges when cut while warm. Materials with memory, or those that have a high resistance to stretch, resist sealing and require additional finishing.

SOFT SPLINT MATERIALS

Soft, flexible materials such as cotton duck, neoprene, knit elastics, and plastic-impregnated materials may be used alone or in combination with metal or plastic stays to fabricate semiflexible splints. These materials allow for the fabrication of splints that permit partial motion around a joint, yet still limit or protect the part. Semiflexible splints are sometimes used during sporting activities and to assist clients with chronic pain when returning to functional activity. Semiflexible splints are also used for geriatric clients and for clients with arthritis who often cannot tolerate rigid splints.

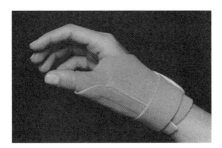

FIGURE 4-30 Flexible thumb splint provides support and allows midrange movement.

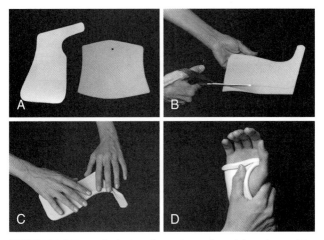

FIGURE 4-31 A, Pattern for single-surface cock-up splint on *left* requires precision for a proper fit. Pattern on *right* for circumferential splint does not need precise fit because material stretches and overlaps to achieve proper size. **B,** Support material on table to prevent stretching and cut with long strokes of scissors. **C,** Fold edges of material and gently press flat to create thin, smooth edges that distribute pressure better. **D,** Gently support the wrist at all times to achieve proper fit.

Suspension Sling

Suspension arm devices are suspended from above the head, generally on an overhead suspension rod that is most often attached to a wheelchair. They can also be attached to regular chairs, a child's highchair, a body jacket, and even an overhead track used for walking clients. Without the suspension rod, they are also attached to over-bed frames to allow the client to use the device while in bed.

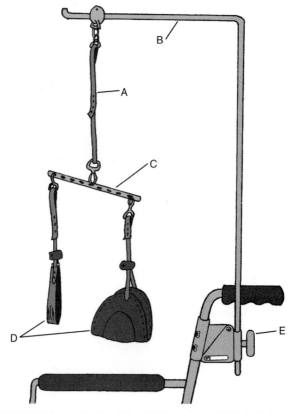

FIGURE 4-32 Suspension sling. **A,** Strap. **B,** Suspension rod. **C,** Horizontal bar (adjustable balance bar). **D,** Wrist and elbow suspension slings. **E,** Adjustable suspension mount. (Adapted from Occupational Therapy Department, Rancho Los Amigos Hospital, Downey, Calif.)

Mobile Arm Support

Mobile arm supports (MASs) are mechanical devices that support the weight of the arm and provide assistance to shoulder and elbow motions through a linkage of ball-bearing joints. They are used for persons with weakness of the shoulder and elbow that affects their ability to position the hand. Mobile arm supports are or have been known by other names such as ball-bearing feeder, ball-bearing arm support, balanced forearm orthosis (BFO), and arm positioner.

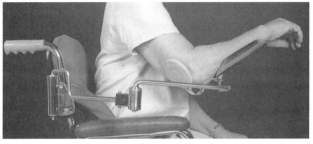

FIGURE 4-33 Traditional mobile arm support set up on a wheelchair. (Courtesy Paul Weinreich, Rancho Los Amigos National Rehabilitation Center, Downey, Calif.)

Neurologic Considerations for Traditional Sensorimotor Approaches to Intervention

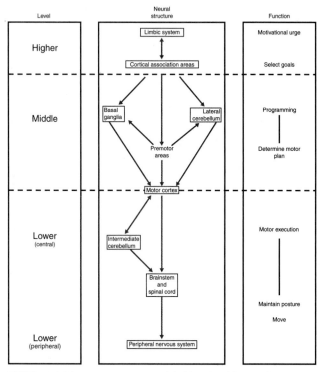

FIGURE 4-34 Schematic representation of the hierarchy of the neural structures involved in motor control. The *left column,* hierarchical level, and the *right column,* indicate the major function of the neural structures shown in the *center column* during motor performance. (Adapted from Cheney PD: Role of cerebral cortex in voluntary movements: A review. *Phys Ther* 65:624-635, 1985.)

The CNS structures involved with movement can be grouped functionally into higher, middle, and lower levels. The higher level consists of the limbic system and association areas, where the motivation for action is generated. The sensorimotor areas, along with the basal ganglia and cerebellum, form the middle level, and the lower level consists of the nuclei in the brainstem and spinal cord. Under normal circumstances, an individual's repertoire of motor activity is varied and complex, meeting unique task and environmental demands. After damage to the central nervous system (CNS) regions involved with movement, the coordinated efforts between the various levels of motor control are disrupted and the motor response may be limited or stereotyped. Traditional sensorimotor approaches to intervention can be viewed as targeting the middle sensorimotor level, the motor planning–strategy formulation process, and the lower level execution process, with the aim of reintegrating, as far as possible, a complete motor control hierarchy. It easily can be seen that a motor relearning program should also be cognitively oriented and targeted toward achieving a goal or occupational task and include all three levels of CNS function related to motor control. This represents the inherent limitation of the traditional sensorimotor approaches. These approaches do not actively engage the client's volitional intent or motivation to perform a motor act. The limitations of traditional sensorimotor approaches must be carefully considered prior to selecting this form of intervention for the client.

The foundational premise of these traditional sensorimotor approaches posits that clients need to be taught motor strategies or compensatory mechanisms to adapt to the deficits produced by a lesion. Compensatory mechanisms and the shaping of motor programs are brought about by the use of sensory inputs. The sensorimotor approaches use sensory stimulation to elicit specific movement patterns. Early in the intervention phase, the emphasis is on the use of external sensory stimuli. Once a movement response is obtained, to reinforce and strengthen the response, the focus shifts to the use of intrinsic sensory information, which thereby encourages voluntary motor control.

The four traditional sensorimotor intervention approaches historically used by occupational therapy (OT) practitioners are the

Rood approach, Brunnstrom (movement therapy) approach, proprioceptive neuromuscular facilitation approach (PNF), and neurodevelopmental (Bobath or NDT) approach. These approaches, developed in the 1950s and 1960s, all have their theoretical basis in the reflex and hierarchical models of motor control. Although more contemporary models are currently being used to guide intervention with clients who demonstrate CNS dysfunction, an understanding of these traditional approaches is warranted to appreciate their contributions to clinical practice and to recognize the appropriate application of these approaches in selected populations.

Overview: The Traditional Sensorimotor Intervention Approaches

ROOD APPROACH

Key components of the Rood approach are the use of sensory stimulation to evoke a motor response and the use of developmental postures to promote changes in muscle tone. Sensory stimulation is applied to muscles and joints to elicit a specific motor response. Stimulation has the potential to have an inhibitory or a facilitatory effect on muscle tone. Types of sensory stimulation described by Rood include the use of slow rolling, neutral warmth, deep pressure, tapping, and prolonged stretch. Examples of how this stimulation may be applied include tapping over a muscle belly to facilitate (increase) muscle tone and applying deep pressure to a muscle's tendinous insertion to elicit an inhibitory (decreased) effect.

BRUNNSTROM (MOVEMENT THERAPY) APPROACH

In the Brunnstrom approach, emphasis is placed on facilitating the progress of the individual by promotion of movement from reflexive to volitional. In the early stages of recovery, this may include the incorporation of reflexes and associated reactions to change tone and achieve movement. For example, to generate reflexive movement in the arm, resistance may be applied to one side of the body to increase muscle tone on the opposite side. This technique is applied until the client demonstrates volitional control over the movement pattern.

PROPRIOCEPTIVE NEUROMUSCULAR FACILITATION APPROACH

Major emphasis in this approach is on the developmental sequencing of movement and the balanced interplay between agonist and antagonist in producing volitional movement. PNF describes mass movement patterns, which are diagonal in nature, for the limbs and trunk. Intervention strategies use these patterns to promote movement. The use of sensory stimulation, including tactile, auditory, and visual inputs, is also actively incorporated into treatment to promote a motor response.

NEURODEVELOPMENTAL TREATMENT APPROACH

The primary objectives of neurodevelopmental treatment are to normalize muscle tone, inhibit primitive reflexes, and facilitate normal postural reactions. Improving the quality of movement and helping clients relearn normal movement patterns are key objectives of this approach. To achieve these objectives, therapists use a number of techniques, including handling techniques, weight bearing over the affected limb, positions that encourage the use of both sides of the body, and avoidance of any sensory input that may adversely affect muscle tone. In clinical practice today, many of these techniques and strategies are used within the context of purposeful activities.

TABLE 4-1 Comparison of Key Treatment Strategies Used in the Traditional Sensorimotor Approaches

Key Treatment Strategies	Rood Approach	Treatment Approach		
		Brunnstrom Approach (Movement Therapy)	Proprioceptive Neuromuscular Approach	Neurodevelopmental Treatment
Sensory stimulation used to evoke a motor response	Yes (uses direct application of sensory stimuli to muscles and joints)	Yes (movement occurs in response to sensory stimuli)	Yes (tactile, auditory, visual sensory stimuli promote motor responses)	Yes (abnormal muscle tone occurs, partly because of abnormal sensory experiences)
Reflexive movement used as a precursor for volitional movement	Yes (reflexive movement achieved initially through application of sensory stimuli)	Yes (move patient along continuum of reflexive to volitional movement patterns)	Yes (volitional movements can be assisted by reflexive supported postures)	No
Treatment directed toward influencing muscle tone	Yes (sensory stimuli used to inhibit or facilitate tone)	Yes (postures, sensory stimuli used to inhibit or facilitate tone)	Yes (movement patterns used to normalize tone)	Yes (handling techniques and postures can inhibit or facilitate muscle tone)
Developmental patterns and sequences used for development of motor skills	Yes (ontogenic motor patterns used to develop motor skills)	Yes (flexion and extension synergies; proximal to distal return)	Yes (patterns used to facilitate proximal to distal motor control)	Yes
Conscious attention directed toward movement	No	Yes	Yes	Yes
Treatment directly emphasizes development of skilled movements for task performance	No	No	No	Yes

TABLE 4-2 Motor Recovery After Cerebrovascular Accident*

Stage	Characteristics Leg	Arm	Hand
1	Flaccidity	Flaccidity; inability to perform any movements	No hand function
2	Spasticity develops; minimal voluntary movements	Beginning development of spasticity; limb synergies or some of their components begin to appear as associated reactions	Gross grasp beginning; minimal finger flexion possible
3	Spasticity peaks; flexion and extension synergy present; hip-knee-ankle flexion in sitting and standing	Spasticity increasing; synergy patterns or some of their components can be performed voluntarily	Gross grasp, hook grasp possible; no release
4	Knee flexion past 90 degrees in sitting, with foot sliding backward on floor; dorsiflexion with heel on floor and knee flexed to 90 degrees	Spasticity declining; movement combinations deviating from synergies now possible	Gross grasp present; lateral prehension developing; small amount of finger extension and some thumb movement possible
5	Knee flexion with hip extended in standing; ankle dorsiflexion with hip and knee extended	Synergies no longer dominant; more movement combinations deviating from synergies performed with greater ease	Palmar prehension, spherical and cylindrical grasp and release possible
6	Hip abduction in sitting or standing; reciprocal internal and external rotation of hip combined with inversion and eversion of ankle in sitting	Spasticity absent except when performing rapid movements; isolated joint movements performed with ease	All types of prehension, individual finger motion, and full range of voluntary extension possible

*Recovery of hand function is variable and may not parallel the six recovery stages of the arm.
From Brunnstrom S: *Movement therapy in hemiplegia*, New York, Harper & Row, 1970.

Motor Learning

Motor learning is the acquisition and modification of learned movement patterns over time. It involves cognitive and perceptual processes to code various motor programs. Motor learning involves practice and experience, which leads to permanent changes in the person's ability to produce movement sufficient to the demands of occupational performance. Motor control is the outcome of motor learning and involves the ability to produce purposeful movements of the extremities and postural adjustments in response to activity and environmental demands.

Constraint-induced movement therapy (CIMT), or forced use, is a therapeutic strategy designed to promote functional use of the hemiparetic upper extremity and has been credited with speeding up the cortical map reorganization process in nonhuman primates and in humans. CIMT is also based on the principles of dynamic systems theory and a task-oriented approach to motor control acquisition. In other methods of stroke rehabilitation, clients learn to use the more functional, or less involved, upper extremity for daily activities. This treatment approach may foster learned nonuse of the more involved upper extremity. Learned nonuse is a phenomenon in which the individual neglects to use the affected, or more involved, extremity because of the extreme difficulty coordinating movement after the onset of a stroke, brain injury, or other neurologic condition.

Shaping procedures are behavioral techniques that approach a desired motor outcome in small, successive increments. Shaping strategies allow subjects to experience successful gains in performance with relatively small amounts of motor improvement.

To determine whether a subject meets inclusion criteria for CIMT, a telephone screening protocol is often administered. Many research studies use a CIMT protocol that contains typical inclusion criteria for use of this therapeutic strategy. These criteria can include the following: (1) a first-time CVA that occurred more than 1 year ago; (2) not currently receiving therapeutic intervention; (3) a score of more than 44 on the Berg balance test or limited balance problems requiring an assistive device for mobility in clients who have had a full-time caregiver to assist with any balance issues; (4) ability to move the affected arm in 45 degrees of shoulder flexion and abduction, 90 degrees of elbow flexion and extension, 20 degrees of wrist extension, and 10 degrees of extension at metacarpal phalanges and interphalanges, as determined by the client's available active ROM (Fig. 4-35); (5) no significant cognitive impairments as demonstrated by a Mini-Mental State Examination score of at least 22, or another type of cognitive test; (6) no preexisting comorbidities that might interfere with mobility or function; (7) limited spasticity (score of 0 or 1) as measured by the modified Ashworth scale; and (8) the ability

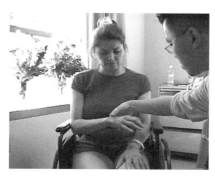

FIGURE 4-35 The patient is asked to demonstrate active wrist and finger extension in her dominant right hand. She is able to achieve 20 degrees of wrist extension and 10 degrees of finger extension (at the metacarpal phalanges) from a flexed position. (Courtesy Remy Chu, OTR/L.)

to identify an individual or caregiver who could assist with the home program.

A battery of assessments are typically administered with all clients included in a CIMT treatment program. Results from these assessments are used to test certain research hypotheses, whereas other assessments are used for diagnostic purposes or to generate new hypotheses. Some typical assessments include the Wolf Motor Function Test (WMFT) and the Motor Activity Log (MAL).

The WMFT consists of 15 motor items that examine contributions from the distal and proximal muscles of the arm. The tasks in this assessment are sequenced from proximal to distal and gross to fine motor. Most tasks are completed with the subject seated in a chair. Standard tasks such as lifting the forearm to the table, reaching for an object, or lifting a pencil are rated on a scale from 0 (does not attempt with weaker arm) to 5 (movement appears normal) and the time to complete the task is measured; Fig. 4-36). The WMFT uses a grid or template that is taped to the desk to specify standardized measurements. The WMFT is administered before the intervention, immediately after the intervention, and at a designated follow-up time.

The MAL was developed for the purpose of assessing activities attempted outside the clinical setting. The MAL is a self-report, 30-item instrument administered in an interview format. Subjects are asked to rate their performance on each activity reported and

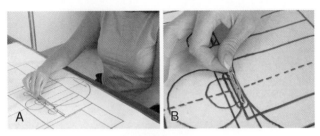

FIGURE 4-36 The Wolf Motor Function Test includes standard tasks such as lifting the forearm to the table and reaching for an object.

emphasis is placed on the client's functional use of the hemiparetic upper extremity in his or her home environment. The assessment is administered approximately 10 times throughout the course of CIMT intervention. The instrument consists of specific functional activities, such as turning on a light switch or opening a drawer. The amount of functional use of the more involved upper extremity is rated by the participant from 0 (never used) to 5 (involved arm used the same as it was before the stroke). The quality of movement (how well) is also self-rated from 0 (not used) to 5 (normal movement).

Intervention Applications

Cerebrovascular Accident/Stroke

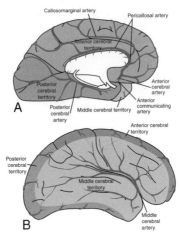

FIGURE 5-1 Blood supply to brain. Middle cerebral, anterior cerebral, and posterior cerebral arteries supply blood to cerebral hemispheres. **A,** Medial surface. **B,** Lateral surface. (From Nolte J: *The human brain: An introduction to its functional anatomy,* 6th ed. Philadelphia, Elsevier, 2009.)

TABLE 5-1 Cerebral Artery Dysfunction: Cortical Involvement and Patterns of Impairment

Artery	Location	Possible Impairments
Middle cerebral artery, upper trunk	Lateral aspect of frontal and parietal lobe	Dysfunction of Either Hemisphere Contralateral hemiplegia, especially of the face and the upper extremity Contralateral hemisensory loss Visual field impairment Poor contralateral conjugate gaze Ideational apraxia Lack of judgment Perseveration Field dependency Impaired organization of behavior Depression Lability Apathy Right Hemisphere Dysfunction Left unilateral body neglect Left unilateral visual neglect Anosognosia Visuospatial impairment Left unilateral motor apraxia Left Hemisphere Dysfunction Bilateral motor apraxia Broca's aphasia Frustration
Middle cerebral artery, lower trunk	Lateral aspect of right temporal and occipital lobes	Dysfunction of Either Hemisphere Contralateral visual field defect Behavioral abnormalities Right Hemisphere Dysfunction Visuospatial dysfunction Left Hemisphere Dysfunction Wernicke's aphasia
Middle cerebral artery, both upper and lower trunks	Lateral aspect of the involved hemisphere	Impairments related to upper and lower trunk dysfunction as listed in previous two sections

Continued

TABLE 5-1 Cerebral Artery Dysfunction: Cortical Involvement and Patterns of Impairment—cont'd

Artery	Location	Possible Impairments
Anterior cerebral artery	Medial and superior aspect of frontal and parietal lobes	Contralateral hemiparesis, greatest in foot Contralateral hemisensory loss, greatest in foot Left unilateral apraxia Inertia of speech or mutism Behavioral disturbances
Internal carotid artery	Combination of middle cerebral artery distribution and anterior cerebral artery	Impairments related to dysfunction of middle and anterior cerebral arteries as listed in previous sections
Anterior choroidal artery, a branch of the internal carotid artery	Globus pallidus, lateral geniculate body, posterior limb of the internal capsule, medial temporal lobe	Hemiparesis of face, arm, and leg Hemisensory loss Hemianopsia
Posterior cerebral artery	Medial and inferior aspects of right temporal and occipital lobes, posterior corpus callosum and penetrating arteries to midbrain and thalamus	Dysfunction of Either Side Homonymous hemianopsia Visual agnosia (visual object agnosia, prosopagnosia, color agnosia) Memory impairment Occasional contralateral numbness Right Side Dysfunction Cortical blindness Visuospatial impairment Impaired left-right discrimination Left Side Dysfunction Finger agnosia Anomia Agraphia Acalculia Alexia
Basilar artery proximal	Pons	Quadriparesis Bilateral asymmetric weakness Bulbar or pseudobulbar paralysis (bilateral paralysis of face, palate, pharynx, neck, or tongue) Paralysis of eye abductors Nystagmus Ptosis Cranial nerve abnormalities Diplopia Dizziness Occipital headache Coma

TABLE 5-1 Cerebral Artery Dysfunction: Cortical Involvement and Patterns of Impairment—cont'd

Artery	Location	Possible Impairments
Basilar artery distal	Midbrain, thalamus, and caudate nucleus	Papillary abnormalities Abnormal eye movements Altered level of alertness Coma Memory loss Agitation Hallucination
Vertebral artery	Lateral medulla and cerebellum	Dizziness Vomiting Nystagmus Pain in ipsilateral eye and face Numbness in face Clumsiness of ipsilateral limbs Hypotonia of ipsilateral limbs Tachycardia Gait ataxia
Systemic hypoperfusion	Watershed region on lateral side of hemisphere, hippocampus, and surrounding structures in medial temporal lobe	Coma Dizziness Confusion Decreased concentration Agitation Memory impairment Visual abnormalities caused by disconnection from frontal eye fields Simultanagnosia Impaired eye movements Weakness of shoulder and arm Gait ataxia

From Arnadottir G: Impact of neurobehavioral deficits of activities of daily living. In Gillen G (ed): *Stroke rehabilitation: A function-based approach,* 3rd ed. St. Louis, Elsevier/Mosby, 2011, pp.

TABLE 5-2 Cerebrovascular Dysfunction in Noncortical Areas: Patterns of Impairment

Location	Possible Impairments
Anterolateral thalamus, either side	Minor contralateral motor abnormalities Long latency period Slowness Right side: Visual neglect Left side: Aphasia
Lateral thalamus	Contralateral hemisensory symptoms Contralateral limb ataxia
Bilateral thalamus	Memory impairment Behavioral abnormalities Hypersomnolence
Internal capsule or basis pontis	Pure motor stroke
Posterior thalamus	Numbness or decreased sensibility of face and arm Choreic movements Impaired eye movements Hypersomnolence Decreased consciousness Decreased alertness Right side: Visual neglect, anosognosia, visuospatial abnormalities Left side: Aphasia, jargon aphasia, good comprehension of speech, paraphasia, anomia
Caudate	Dysarthria Apathy Restlessness Agitation Confusion Delirium Lack of initiative Poor memory Contralateral hemiparesis Ipsilateral conjugate deviation of the eyes
Putamen	Contralateral hemiparesis Contralateral hemisensory loss Decreased consciousness Ipsilateral conjugate gaze Motor impersistence Right side: Visuospatial impairment Left side: Aphasia
Pons	Quadriplegia Coma Impaired eye movement
Cerebellum	Ipsilateral limb ataxia Gait ataxia Vomiting Impaired eye movements

From Arnadottir G: Impact of neurobehavioral deficits of activities of daily living. In Gillen G (ed): *Stroke rehabilitation: A function-based approach*, 3rd ed. St. Louis, Elsevier/Mosby, 2011, pp.

Traumatic Brain Injury

Traumatic brain injury (TBI) is defined as damage to brain tissue caused by an external mechanical force with resultant loss of consciousness, post-traumatic amnesia (PTA), skull fracture, or objective neurologic findings that can be attributed to the traumatic event on the basis of radiologic findings or physical or mental status examination. It is the most common cause of death and disability in young people.

The cause of TBI is closely associated with age and gender. Children younger than 5 years tend to be injured in falls and motor vehicle accidents (MVAs), and by adults inflicting violence. Those between ages 5 and 15 are also injured on bicycles, skateboards, and horses; as pedestrians; and during sports activities. Between ages 15 and 40, high-speed MVAs and motorcycle crashes are the most common causes of TBI. After age 40, the incidence of violence-related injury approaches that of MVAs, particularly in metropolitan areas. Young and middle-aged adult males are 1.5 times more likely to be injured than their female counterparts. The two age groups at highest risk for a TBI are 0- to 4-year olds and 15- to 19-year olds. Older individuals are injured just as often by a fall or during a pedestrian mishap as they are in MVAs. Blasts are a leading cause of TBIs for active duty military personnel in war zones.

Nontraumatic brain injuries include toxicity from drug overdose, chronic substance abuse, carbon monoxide poisoning, or environmental exposure, anoxia from cardiopulmonary arrest or near-drowning, brain abscess, meningitis, and encephalitis from bacteria, viruses, acquired immunodeficiency syndrome (AIDS), fungi, or parasites, nutritional deficiencies, genetic and congenital disorders, chronic epilepsy, and degenerative diseases such as dementia.

Focal brain injury is caused by a direct blow to the head after collision with an external object or fall, a penetrating injury resulting from a weapon, and the collision of the brain with the inner tables of the skull. The bones of the face or skull may or may not be fractured. Common findings of focal injury that results from falls include intracerebral and brain surface contusions, particularly in the inferior and dorsolateral frontal lobes, anterior and medial temporal lobes and, less commonly, the inferior cerebellum. Assaults and missile wounds can occur anywhere in the brain, depending on the direction of force. Other surface areas of the brain, including those not directly below the blow to the head, can also suffer contusions as a result of the collision of the brain with the inner tables of the skull. The directly injured area is referred to as the coup and the site of the indirect injury is known as the contre coup.

If there are injuries to the coverings of the brain, especially the dura, pia, and arachnoid, other focal hemorrhages occur. Epidural hematomas (EDHs) are associated with skull fractures in adults with disruption of the integrity of the meningeal arteries; children may have arterial disruption with or without skull fracture. Individuals with an EDH may be initially alert after the blow to the skull; as the hematoma develops between the skull and the dura, it can cause pressure on underlying brain tissue (secondary injury), with rapid deterioration in mental and physical status. Prompt recognition and neurosurgical treatment can save lives and limit morbidity.

Subdural hematomas (SDHs) occur between the dura and the brain surface through tearing of bridging veins. The rate of hemorrhage is often slower than that of an EDH because venous bleeding is more gradual than arterial bleeding. SDH may occur just as frequently on the side of the head opposite the direct blow; therefore, an EDH can occur on one side of the brain adjacent to the trauma, with an SDH on the other. SDHs tend to spread around the entire surface of one hemisphere or, less commonly, in the posterior fossa. Acute SDH is diagnosed within 48 hours of injury, subacute SDH within 2 to 14 days after injury, and chronic SDH after 2 weeks. The fall or blow to the head in subacute or chronic SDH may have occurred days before the person arrives at the hospital, with symptoms typical of mental status changes. The urgency regarding SDH treatment depends on the clinical condition of the individual and the degree of mass of adjacent brain tissue observed on radiologic findings.

With multifocal and diffuse brain injuries, there may be sudden deceleration of the body and head, with variable forces transmitted to the surface and deeper portions of the brain. Motor vehicle, bicycle, and skateboard crashes are typical causative factors, but falls from a high surface or off a horse or bull can also result in multifocal and diffuse injuries.

Intracerebral hemorrhage (ICH) is almost always present with missile wounds as focal injury and is common after falls and assaults. Within the first week after the TBI, particularly in clients with blood-clotting abnormalities, ICH may appear on follow-up CT scans. With high-speed deceleration injury, multiple small, deep intracerebral hemorrhages occur throughout the neuraxis: on high-resolution CT or MRI scans, they are typically visible at the junction between the gray and white matter, basal ganglia, corpus callosum, midbrain, and/or cerebellum.

Subarachnoid (SAH) and intraventricular hemorrhages (IVH) occur when the pia or arachnoid are torn. SAH caused by trauma is less frequently associated with vasospasms than SAH caused by aneurysm rupture. A large IVH can block cerebral spinal fluid (CSF) flow, resulting in acute hydrocephalus. Thus, clinical evaluation of the possibility of a ruptured aneurysm that causes brain dysfunction, which may result from a fall or motor vehicle crash, is important with either of these entities.

Diffuse axonal injuries (DAIs) are a prototypical lesion caused by rapid deceleration. The degree of injury may vary from primary axonotomy, with complete disruption of the nerve, to axonal dysfunction, wherein the structural integrity of the nerve remains but there is loss of ability to transmit normally along neuronal pathways. The clinical severity of DAI is measured by the depth and length of coma (i.e., the time from the onset of injury until the individual performs purposeful activity) and associated signs such as pupillary abnormalities.

TABLE 5-3   Glasgow Coma Scale

Examiner's Test	Individual's Response	Assigned Score
Eye opening		
Spontaneous	Opens eyes on own	4
Speech	Opens eyes when asked to in a loud voice	3
Pain	Opens eyes when pinched	2
Pain	Does not open eyes	1
Best motor response		
Commands	Follows simple commands	6
Pain	Pulls examiner's hand away when pinched	5
Pain	Pulls a part of body away when pinched by examiner	4
Pain	Flexes body inappropriately to pain (decorticate posturing)	3
Pain	Body becomes rigid in an extended position when examiner pinches victim (decerebrate posturing)	2
Pain	Has no motor response to pinch	1
Verbal response (talking)		
Speech	Carries on a conversation correctly and tells examiner where and who he or she is and the month and year	5
Speech	Seems confused or disoriented	4
Speech	Talks so examiner can understand but makes no sense	3
Speech	Makes sounds that examiner can't understand	2
Speech	Makes no noise	1

From Rosenthal M: *Rehabilitation of the head-injured adult*, Philadelphia, FA Davis, 1984.

TABLE 5-4   Duration of Post-Traumatic Amnesia (PTA) and Severity of Injury

PTA Duration	Severity
Less than 5 min	Very mild
5 to 60 min	Mild
1 to 24 hr	Moderate
1 to 7 days	Severe
1 to 4 wk	Very severe
More than 4 wk	Extremely severe

From Rosenthal M: *Rehabilitation of the head-injured adult.* Philadelphia, FA Davis, 1984.

BOX 5-1 Rancho Los Amigos (RLA) Levels of Cognitive Functioning

I. No response. Individual appears to be in a deep sleep and is completely unresponsive to any stimuli presented to him or her.

II. Generalized response. The individual reacts inconsistently and nonpurposefully to stimuli in a nonspecific manner. Responses are limited in nature and are often the same, regardless of the stimulus presented. Responses may be physiologic changes, gross body movements, or vocalization. Often, the earliest response is to deep pain. Responses are likely to be delayed.

III. Localized response. The individual reacts specifically but inconsistently to stimuli. Responses are directly related to the type of stimulus presented, as in turning the head toward a sound or focusing on an object presented. The individual may withdraw an extremity or vocalize when presented with a painful stimulus. He or she may follow simple commands in an inconsistent, delayed manner, such as in closing the eyes, squeezing, or extending an extremity. After the external stimulus is removed, the individual may lie quietly. He or she may also show a vague awareness of self and body by responding to discomfort by pulling at a nasogastric (NG) tube or catheter or resisting restraints. The individual may show bias by responding to some persons (especially family, friends) but not to others.

IV. Confused-agitated. The individual is in a heightened state of activity with a severely decreased ability to process information. He or she is detached from the present and responds primarily to his or her own internal confusion. Behavior is frequently bizarre and nonpurposeful relative to the immediate environment. The individual may cry out or scream out of proportion to stimuli even after removal and may show aggressive behavior, attempt to remove restraints or tubes, or crawl out of bed in a purposeful manner. The individual does not, however, discriminate among persons or objects and is unable to cooperate directly with treatment effort. Verbalization is frequently incoherent and inappropriate to the environment. Confabulation may be present; the individual may be euphoric or hostile. Thus, gross attention is very short and selective attention is often nonexistent. Being unaware of present events, the individual lacks short-term recall and may be reacting to past events. He or she is unable to perform self-care (e.g., feeding, dressing) without maximal assistance. If not disabled physically, the individual may perform motor activities as in sitting, reaching, and ambulating but as part of the agitated state and not as a purposeful act or on request.

V. Confused, inappropriate, nonagitated. The individual appears alert and is able to respond to simple commands fairly consistently. However, with increased complexity of commands or lack of any external structure, responses are nonpurposeful, random, or at best fragmented toward any desired goal. The individual may show agitated behavior, not on an internal basis (as in level IV) but rather as a result of external stimuli and usually out of proportion to the stimulus. He or she has gross attention to the environment but is highly distractible and lacks the ability to focus attention to a specific task without frequent redirection back to it. With structure, the individual may be able to converse on a social, automatic level for short periods of time. Verbalization is often inappropriate; confabulation may be triggered by present events. Memory is severely impaired, with confusion of past and present in his or her reaction to ongoing activity. The individual lacks initiation with regard to functional tasks and often shows inappropriate use of objects without external direction. He or she may be able to perform previously learned tasks when they are structured for him or her, but the individual is unable to learn new information. He or she responds best to self, body, comfort—and often family members. The individual can usually perform self-care activities with assistance and may accomplish feeding with maximal supervision. Management on the ward is often a problem if the individual is physically mobile, because he or she may wander off randomly or with the vague intention of going home.

VI. Confused-appropriate. The individual shows goal-directed behavior but is dependent on external input for direction. The response to discomfort is appropriate, and the individual is able to tolerate unpleasant stimuli (e.g., NG tube) when the need is explained. The individual follows simple directions consistently and shows carryover for tasks that have

Continued

BOX 5-1 Rancho Los Amigos (RLA) Levels of Cognitive Functioning—cont'd

been relearned (such as self-care). He or she is at least supervised with old learning and is unable to assist maximally for new learning, with little or no carryover. Responses may be incorrect because of memory problems, but they are appropriate to the situation. Responses may be delayed, and the individual shows a decreased ability to process information, with little or no anticipation or prediction of events. Past memories show more depth and detail than recent memory. The individual may show beginning awareness of his or her situation by realizing that he or she doesn't know an answer. The individual no longer wanders and is inconsistently oriented to time and place. Selective attention to tasks may be impaired, especially with difficult tasks and in unstructured settings, but the individual is now functional for common daily activities (30 minutes with structure). He or she shows at least vague recognition of some staff and has increased awareness of self, family, and basic needs (e.g., food), again in an appropriate manner, as in contrast to level V.

VII. Automatic-appropriate. The individual appears appropriate and oriented within hospital and home settings and goes through the daily routine automatically but is frequently robot-like. The individual has minimal to absent confusion but has shallow recall of what he or she has been doing. He or she shows increased awareness of self, body, family, foods, people, and interaction in the environment. The individual has superficial awareness of, but lacks insight into, his or her condition; demonstrates decreased judgment and problem solving; and lacks realistic planning for the future. He or she shows carryover for new learning but at a decreased rate. He or she requires at least minimal supervision for learning and for safety purposes and is independent in self-care activities and supervised in home and community skills for safety. With structure, the individual is able to initiate tasks in social and recreational activities in which he or she now has interest. Judgment remains impaired, such that the individual is unable to drive a car. Prevocational or avocational evaluation and counseling may be indicated.

VIII. Purposeful and appropriate. The individual is alert and oriented, is able to recall and integrate past and recent events, and is aware of and responsive to his or her culture. He or she shows carryover for new learning if it is acceptable to him or her and his or her life role. The individual needs no supervision after activities are learned within his or her physical capabilities. He or she is independent in home and community skills, including driving. Vocational rehabilitation, to determine ability to return as a contributor to society (perhaps in a new capacity), is indicated. The individual may continue to show a decreased ability, relative to premorbid abilities, in reasoning, tolerance for stress, judgment in emergencies, or unusual circumstances. His or her social, emotional, and intellectual capacities may continue to be at a decreased level but are functional for society.

The following additional RLA levels are used at some outpatient facilities to identify higher functioning clients.

Level IX: Purposeful, Appropriate: Standby Assistance on Request

- Independently shifts back and forth between tasks and completes them accurately for at least 2 consecutive hours
- Uses assistive memory devices to recall daily schedule and "to do" lists, and record critical information for later use with assistance when requested
- Initiates and carries out steps to complete familiar personal, household, work and leisure tasks independently and unfamiliar personal, household, work and leisure tasks with assistance when requested
- Aware of and acknowledges impairments and disabilities when they interfere with task completion; takes appropriate corrective action but requires standby assist to anticipate a problem before it occurs and take action to avoid it
- Able to think about consequences of decisions or actions with assistance when requested
- Accurately estimates abilities but requires standby assistance to adjust to task demands
- Acknowledges others' needs and feelings and responds appropriately with standby assistance
- Depression may continue.
- May be easily irritable
- May have low frustration tolerance
- Able to self-monitor appropriateness of social interaction with standby assistance

BOX 5-1 Rancho Los Amigos (RLA) Levels of Cognitive Functioning—cont'd

Level X: Purposeful, Appropriate: Modified Independent

- Able to handle multiple tasks simultaneously in all environments but may require periodic breaks
- Able to procure, create, and maintain own assistive memory devices independently
- Independently initiates and carries out steps to complete familiar and unfamiliar personal, household, community, work and leisure tasks but may require more than usual amount of time and/or compensatory strategies to complete them
- Anticipates impact of impairments and disabilities on ability to complete daily living tasks and takes action to avoid problems before they occur but may require more than usual amount of time and/or compensatory strategies
- Able to think about consequences of decisions or actions independently but may require more than usual amount of time and/or compensatory strategies to select the appropriate decision or action
- Accurately estimates abilities and independently adjusts to task demands
- Able to recognize the needs and feelings of others and automatically respond in appropriate manner
- Periodic periods of depression may occur.
- Irritability and low frustration tolerance when sick, fatigued and/or under emotional stress
- Social interaction behavior is consistently appropriate.

Adapted from Rancho Los Amigos Medical Center, Adult brain injury service: Original scale, levels of cognitive functioning. Rancho Los Amigos Medical Center, Downey, Calif, 1980.

TABLE 5-5 Motor Signs

Motor Sign	Lesion Localization	Clinical Characteristics	Interventions
Decerebrate rigidity	Midbrain, pons, diencephalon	Extended internally rotated shoulders; extended elbows; flexed wrists, fingers; extended internally rotated hips, extended knees, ankle plantar flexion, inversion; increased rigidly when awake	Positioning, ROM, neuromuscular blocks and early casting
Decorticate rigidity	Cortical white matter, internal capsule, thalamus, cerebral peduncle, basal ganglia	Internally rotated shoulder; flexed elbow, wrists, fingers; extended internally rotated hips; knee flexion; ankle plantar flexion, inversion; increased rigidity when awake	Positioning, ROM, neuromuscular blocks and early casting
Bruxism		Persistent jaw clenching, teeth grinding ± temporomandibular dislocation or subluxation	Neuromuscular blocks, oral orthotics
Spasticity	Upper motor neuron syndrome (UMN); cortical spinal pathways	Velocity-dependent resistance, hyperreflexia, clonus, muscle shortening; present in face, neck, trunk, limbs; worse when awake and with effort	Bed, chair positioning, ROM, weight bearing, neuromuscular blocks, inhibitive casting, enteral and intrathecal medications, tendon releases, relaxation techniques
Rigidity and bradykinesia; "parkinsonism"	Substantia nigra; extrapyramidal pathways; also with medications that block dopamine	Velocity-independent resistance; "lead pipe," "cog-wheeling" worse when awake	Positioning, ROM, functional activities, medications
Torticollis		Dystonic posture of neck; spasticity and or contracture of sternocleidomastoid, splenius muscles	Positioning, modalities and ROM, medications, neuromuscular blocks
Myoclonus	Variable	Abrupt, shocklike involuntary jerks in large (limb) or small muscles when sleep or awake	Medications, neuromuscular blocks
Tremor	Variable	Involuntary rhythmic oscillations while awake	Weighted devices, weight bearing, medications, neuromuscular blocks, appropriate assistive devices

Dystonia	Variable	Dynamic contraction and relaxation of muscles with slow, writhing or repetitive twisting movements or sustained contortions; usually distal limb(s)	Positioning, ROM, neuromuscular blocks, medications appropriate assistive devices
Athetosis	Basal ganglia, medications with dopamine effect	Slow sinuous movements of face, tongue, or limbs	Relaxation techniques, taper offending medications
Chorea	Contralateral neostriatum thalamus	Involuntary dancelike or jerky movements without rhythmic pattern; distal	Medications
Hemiballismus, ballismus	Contralateral subthalamic nucleus, thalamus, cerebellum	Sudden irregular flinging movements starting hip or shoulder, occasionally facial or oral ± rotator component worse with arousal or excitement; absent in sleep	Medications
Tics	Variable	Sudden stereotypic coordinated automatic movements or vocalizations while awake	Medications, behavioral management, relaxation techniques
Pseudobulbar athetoid syndrome	Bilateral pyramidal tract	Postural dystonia with fragmentary athetosis ± bradykinesia; often preserved intellect, personality	Positioning, appropriate assistive devices

Data from Mayer NH, Keenan MAE, Esquenzi A: Limbs with restricted or excessive motion after traumatic brain injury. In Rosenthal M (ed): *Rehabilitation of the adult and child with traumatic brain injury*, 3rd ed. Philadelphia, FA Davis, 1999; Mayer NH: Choosing upper limb muscles for focal intervention after traumatic brain injury. *J Head Trauma Rehabil* 19:119-142, 2004; and Zafonte R, Elovic E, Lombard L: Acute care management of post-TBI spasticity. *J Head Trauma Rehabil* 19:89-100, 2004.

Lower Level Individuals

EVALUATION

Clients emerging from coma and at the beginning stages of the injury (Rancho Los Amigos levels I to III) may exhibit minimal arousal and limited purposeful movements. It may be necessary to evaluate these individuals in short sessions and at different times of the day. A quiet environment with minimal distractions will enhance the client's ability to attend to and follow commands. Evaluation includes an assessment of the following:

1. Level of arousal and cognition. Can the client visually attend to the speaker and follow commands such as "Open your mouth" and "Squeeze your eyes closed"? Can he or she communicate through verbalizations, gestures, or eye movements? Does he or she demonstrate purposeful movements such as pulling at vital tubes? How easy or difficult is it to wake the client, and how long can the client stay awake?
2. Vision. Is the client able to scan visually or attend to a person, object, or activity? Can the client maintain eye contact?
3. Sensation. Does the client respond to external stimulation such as pain, temperature, and movement of the joints?
4. Joint range of motion (ROM). Has the client lost ROM in certain joints as a result of decorticate or decerebrate posturing, increased tone or spasticity, contractures, or heterotopic ossification?
5. Motor control. Does the client exhibit decorticate or decerebrate posturing? Is there an increase of tone and spasticity? Is there deceased tone and hypotonicity? Are deep tendon responses present, diminished, or absent? Does the client exhibit the presence of primitive reflexes? Does the client engage in spontaneous motor movements, such as scratching the face?
6. Dysphagia. Does the client handle his or her own secretions, drool, or swallow spontaneously? Does the client demonstrate poor oral-motor control? Answers to these questions provide valuable information as to whether a swallowing evaluation is indicated.

7. Emotional and behavioral factors. Is the client's affect flat or expressive? Are responses such as crying or laughing observed in response to interactions with the rehabilitation team or family members?

INTERVENTION

- Sensory stimulation
- Wheelchair positioning
- Bed positioning
- Splinting and casting
- Dysphagia
- Behavioral and cognition
- Family and caregiver education

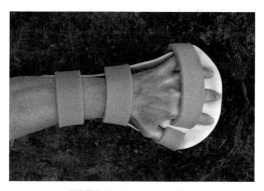

FIGURE 5-2 Antispasticity splint.

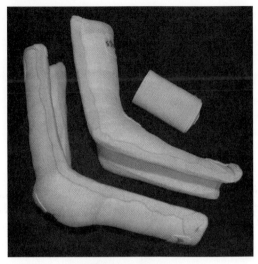

FIGURE 5-3 Spasticity splint.

Intermediate to Higher Level Individual

EVALUATION
- Physical status
- Dysphagia
- Cognition
- Vision
- Perceptual function
- Activities of daily living
- Vocational rehabilitation
- Psychosocial skills

INTERVENTION
- Neuromuscular impairments
- Ataxia
- Cognition
- Vision

- Perception
- Behavioral management
- Dysphagia and self-feeding
- Functional mobility
- Transfers
- Home management
- Community reintegration
- Psychosocial skills
- Substance use
- Discharge planning

TABLE 5-6 Clinical Subtypes of Amyotrophic Lateral Sclerosis

Name	Area of Destruction	Symptoms
Progressive bulbar palsy (PBP; bulbar form)	Corticobulbar tracts and brainstem motor nuclei involved	Dysarthria, dysphagia, facial and tongue weakness, wasting
Progressive spinal muscular atrophy (PMA, PSMA; LMN form)	Lower motor neurons in the spinal cord and sometimes the brainstem	Marked muscle wasting of the limbs, trunk, sometimes the bulbar muscles
Primary lateral sclerosis (PLS; UMN form)*	Destruction of the cortical motor neurons; may involve both corticospinal and corticobulbar regions	Progressive spastic paraparesis

*The World Federation of Neurology Classification of SMAs and other disorders of the motor neurons does not identify PLS as a subtype of ALS. PLS is included here in the list in recognition of the many other articles and books that recognize it as a subtype of ALS.

LMN, Lower motor neuron; UMN, upper motor neuron.

Adapted from Belsh JM, Schiffman PL (eds): *ALS diagnosis and management for the clinician*. Armonk, NY, Futura, 1996; and Guberman A: *An introduction to clinical neurology*, Pathophysiology, Diagnosis, and Treatment. Boston, Little, Brown, 1994.

TABLE 5-7 Amyotrophic Lateral Sclerosis Interventions

Patient Characteristics	Interventions with Focus on Performance Areas of Occupation	Interventions with Focus on Client Factors
Phase I (Independent)		
Stage I Mild weakness Clumsiness Ambulatory Independent with ADLs	Continue normal activities or increase activities if client is sedentary to prevent disuse atrophy and prevent depression. Integrate energy conservation into daily activities, work, and leisure. Provide opportunity for individual to voice concerns (provide psychological support as needed).	Begin ROM program (e.g., stretching, yoga, tai chi). Add strengthening program of gentle resistance exercise to all musculature, using caution to prevent overwork fatigue.
Stage II Moderate, selective weakness Slightly decreased independence in ADLs; for example, difficulty climbing stairs, difficulty raising arms, difficulty buttoning clothing	Assess self-care, work, and leisure skills impaired by loss of function; if patient continues to work, focus on how to adapt tasks with current deficits; assist with balance between work, home, and leisure activities; include significant others in treatment. Use adaptive equipment to facilitate ADLs (e.g., button hook, reacher, built-up utensils, shower seat, grab bar). Integrate hand orthotic use into daily activities. Perform baseline dysphagia evaluation; reevaluate throughout each stage of the disease.	Continue stretching to avoid contractures. Continue cautious strengthening of muscles with manual muscle testing (MMT) grades above F+ (3+). Monitor for overwork fatigue. Consider orthotic support (e.g., ankle-foot orthosis [AFO], wrist or thumb splints—short opponens splint).
Stage III Severe, selective weakness in ankles, wrists, and hands Moderately decreased independence in ADLs Tendency to become easily fatigued with long-distance ambulation Slightly increased respiratory effort	Prescribe manual or power wheelchair with modifications to eventually allow recline or tilt posture with headrest, elevating leg rests, adequate trunk and arm support. Help patient prioritize activities and provide work simplification. Reassess for adaptive equipment needs (universal cuff to eat). Assess and adapt use of communication devices (e.g., regular phone to cordless or speaker phone; pen and paper to computer with adapted typing aid). Provide support if there is loss of employment or other activities; explore alternative activities. Begin discussing need for home modification, such as installing ramps or moving the bedroom to the lowest floor. Provide education regarding the types of bathroom equipment available for energy conservation and safety.	Keep patient physically independent as long as possible through pleasurable activities and walking. Encourage deep breathing exercises, chest stretching, and postural draining if needed.

TABLE 5-7 Amyotrophic Lateral Sclerosis Interventions—cont'd

Patient Characteristics	Interventions with Focus on Performance Areas of Occupation	Interventions with Focus on Client Factors
Phase II (Partially Independent)		
Stage IV Hanging arm syndrome with shoulder pain and sometimes edema in the hand Wheelchair-dependent Severe lower extremity weakness (with or without spasticity) Able to perform some ADLs, but fatigues easily	Evaluate need for arm slings, overhead slings, mobile arm supports for eating, typing, page turning. Prescribe power wheelchair if the patient wants to be independent with mobility; controls must be adaptable from hand to other mode of control. Evaluate need for assistive technology such as environmental control systems, voice-activated computer; augmentative communication device. Help the patient prioritize activities, and consider negotiating roles with significant others. Reinforce the need for home modifications. Reinforce the need for shower seat or transfer tub bench and shower hose. Assist with patient's ability to participate in closure activities, such as writing letters or making tapes for children, completing a life history, and writing a log on household management for family.	If arm supports are not used, provide arm troughs or wheelchair lap tray for wheelchair positioning, wrist cock-up splints for full resting; hand splints may be needed for positioning. Provide pain and spasm management through the following: Heat, massage as indicated to control spasm and pain Antiedema measures Active assisted or passive ROM exercises to the weak joints; caution to support and rotate shoulder during abduction and joint accessory motions Isometric contraction of all musculature to tolerance
Stage V Sever lower extremity weakness Moderate to severe upper extremity weakness Wheelchair dependent Increasingly dependent in ADLs At risk for skin breakdown caused by poor mobility	Instruct family in methods to assist patient with self-care, especially bathing, dressing, and toileting; aim to minimize caregiver's burden and stress. Provide family training to learn proper transfer, positioning principles, and turning techniques. Instruct in use of mechanical lift if needed for transfers out of bed (patients in slings require head support). Adapt and select essential control devices for telephone, stereo, TV, electric hospital bed controls for independent use. Adapt wheelchair for respiratory unit if needed to allow for continued community access.	Instruct family and patient in skin inspection techniques. Instruct in use of electric hospital bed and antipressure device. Adapt wheelchair for respiratory unit if needed; reassess adequacy of wheelchair cushion for pressure relief.

Continued

TABLE 5-7 Amyotrophic Lateral Sclerosis Interventions—cont'd

Patient Characteristics	Interventions with Focus on Performance Areas of Occupation	Interventions with Focus on Client Factors
Phase III (Dependent)		
Stage VI Dependent, with all positioning in bed or wheelchair Completely dependent in ADLs Extreme fatigue	Eating: Evaluate dysphagia, and recommend appropriate diet; therapist may recommend tube feedings if patient is at high risk for aspiration; recommend suction machine for handling secretions and preventing aspiration. Augmentative speech devices may be recommended, in addition to speech therapy.	Continue with passive ROM exercises for all joints Provide sensory stimulation with massage and skin care.

Adapted from Yase Y, Tsubaki T (eds): *Amyotrophic lateral sclerosis: Recent advances in research and treatment*, Amsterdam, Elsevier Science, 1988; and Umphred DA (ed): *Neurologic rehabilitation*, 3rd ed. St. Louis, Mosby, 1995.

TABLE 5-8 Progression of Alzheimer's Disease and Intervention Considerations

Client Characteristics	Intervention Using Occupational Performance	Intervention Using Performance Patterns and Client Factors
Stage I: Very Mild To Mild Cognitive Decline		
Feels loss of control, less spontaneous; may become more anxious and hostile if confronted with losses	Listen to client concerns; collaborate with client in identifying areas that are challenging, and identify associated feelings (depression or anxiety).	Encourage physical exercise and wellness behavior.
Mild problems with memory and less initiative; difficulty with word choice, attention, and comprehension; repetition sometimes necessary; conversation more superficial; mild problems with gnosis or praxis	Begin training the caregiver to serve as case manager.	Help client and caregiver establish a daily routine, and post it in a central place.
Seems socially and physically intact except to intimates; decline in job performance	Provide educational and other resources disease information, support and relaxation, for support groups, or activities for client and caregiver.	Use environmental aids such as calendars, appointment books, adhesive notes, and notebooks to enhance memory and reinforce engagement in occupation.

TABLE 5-8 Progression of Alzheimer's Disease and Intervention Considerations—cont'd

Client Characteristics	Intervention Using Occupational Performance	Intervention Using Performance Patterns and Client Factors
	Identify roles, activity frequency, and configuration; encourage continuation of or increase in enjoyable activities by keeping a log and planning enjoyable activity daily or weekly; use activity or task as a focus in socialization.	Identify appropriate environments, or adapt for activities that are currently challenging.
	Explore meaning of occupations and occupational role changes with client and caregiver.	In teaching new tasks, use auditory, visual, and kinesthetic input, and provide supportive or positive feedback; grade activity for success to decrease anxiety.
	Identify needs, preferences, and goals of the caregiver. Discuss driving skills and plan for future evaluation and restrictions.	During communication training, rehearse with client how to use "I" statements and assertively express self and needs in response to changed ability and the feelings aroused.
		Educate and train caregiver in how to empower client to keep active and facilitate initiation of tasks.
Stage II: Mild to Moderate Decline (problems from stage I are exacerbated)		
Use of denial, labile moods, anxious or hostile at times; excessive passivity and withdrawal in challenging situations; possible development of paranoia	Emphasize to caregiver the importance of environment in managing dementia at home.	Maintain routines and design environmental support (e.g., lists, posters, pictures) and level of assistance for cues to remember daily routine and important events.
Moderate memory loss, with some gaps in personal history and recent or current events; decreased concentration; possible tendency to lose valued objects; difficulty with complex information and problem solving; difficulty learning new tasks; visuospatial deficits more apparent	Analyze and adapt meaningful leisure, home management, and other productive activities so as to allow the client to participate and exert initiation, independence, and control safely.	Avoid tasks involving new learning; help to simplify surroundings and tasks; make objects accessible, establish expectations for object use, simplify instructions, and clarify the meaning of success.

Continued

TABLE 5-8 Progression of Alzheimer's Disease and Intervention Considerations—cont'd

Client Characteristics	Intervention Using Occupational Performance	Intervention Using Performance Patterns and Client Factors
Need for supervision slowly increases; decreased sociability; moderate impairment that are complicated and mild impairment in some ADLs (e.g., finances, shopping, medications, community mobility, cooking complex meals); no longer employed; complicated hobbies dropped	Identify needs, and design ways to adapt and grade activity by simplifying complex tasks; train the caregiver to provide cognitive support (verbally) with the client on IADLs and some ADLs.	Help caregiver interpret behavioral problems by understanding source of frustration and the effects of memory loss on behavior.
	Encourage scrutiny of family structure and resources to respond to increasing need for supervision; consider outside resources (e.g., day care, legal planning, friendly visitor volunteer, public transportation for the disabled).	Maintain socialization, and structure opportunities in which others initiate socialization to ensure satisfying relationships in group activity and other social activities.
		Use reality orientation activities, photo albums, and pictures around the home as a reminder of the past, past competence, and opportunities for socializing.
		Encourage stretching, walking, and other balance activities.

Stage III: Moderate to Moderately Severe Decline In Cognition (problems from stage II are exacerbated; more difficulties involving physical status)

Reduced affect, increased apathy; sleep disturbances; repetitive behaviors; hostile behavior, paranoia, delusions, agitation and violence possible if client becomes overwhelmed	Maintain involvement in meaningful activity and reactivate alternative roles; identify and design tasks in home management activity; client can assist caregiver with design of productive activity related to former work role.	In managing problem behaviors (e.g., assaultive behavior), teach caregivers to identify problem, understand and consider possible precipitants for the behavior (e.g., feelings; antecedent events; who, where, when; medical problem or task; environment; or communication problem), and adapt own behavior or change the environment.

TABLE 5-8 Progression of Alzheimer's Disease and Intervention Considerations—cont'd

Client Characteristics	Intervention Using Occupational Performance	Intervention Using Performance Patterns and Client Factors
Progressive memory loss of well-known material; some past history retained; client unaware of most recent events; disorientation to time and place and sometimes extended family; progressively impaired concentration; deficits in communication severe; apraxia and agnosia more evident	Help caregiver problem solve and recognize degree of need for initiation, verbal cues, physical assistance, and ADLs; provide time orientation; simplify environment.	It is essential to maintain consistent daily routines as a means of facilitating participation in overlearned tasks, maintaining function, and continuing to define the self.
Slowed response, impaired visual and functional spatial orientation	Support socialization at home and with family or in structured settings outside of the home.	Teach family that overlearned tasks are possible but require safe environment; overall, tasks take longer, need to be simplified, and require setup and grading to comprise two steps or less.
Unable to perform most IADLs; in ADLs, assistance eventually needed with toileting, hygiene, eating, and dressing; beginning signs of urinary and fecal incontinence; wandering behavior	Ensure safety in the home and other environments by making adaptations suited to level of client functioning (e.g., alarms, restricted use of heating devices and sharps, cabinet latches, ID bracelet, visual cues for item location, and visual camouflaging).	Make further environmental adaptations to compensate for perceptual deficits and ensure safe mobility.
		Rehearse and review names of family and others, using pictures Encourage standby or assisted ambulation, stretching, and exercise on a regular basis. In new environments, cue and assist client in navigation, and provide more light and pictorial representations to cue.

Stage IV: Severe Cognitive Decline and Moderate to Severe Physical Decline

Adapted from Baum C: Addressing the needs of the cognitively impaired elderly from a family policy perspective. *Am J Occup Ther* 45:594-606, 1991; Morscheck P: Introduction: An overview of Alzheimer's disease and long-term care. *Pride Inst J Long Term Health Care* 3:4-10, 1984; Glickstein J: *Therapeutic interventions in Alzheimer's disease.* Gaithersburg, Md, Aspen, 1997; Gwyther L, Matteson M: Care for the caregivers. *J Gerontol Nurs* 9:93-95, 1983.

TABLE 5-9 Progression of Symptoms in PD

Stage	Symptoms	OT Management
1	Unilateral tremor, micrographia, poor endurance for previous occupations, fatigue	Work evaluation if client is employed; work simplification for work and home settings; develop the habit of taking frequent rest breaks; use of utensils with enlarged handles
2	Bilateral motor disturbances, mild rigidity reported, difficulties with simultaneous tasks, difficulties with executive function	Energy conservation techniques related to ADLs; develop a daily flexibility exercises focused on trunk rotation; driving assessment and alternatives for community mobility; use of task analysis to structure sequential tasks
3	Balance problems with delayed reactions, difficulties with skilled sequential tasks	Environmental modifications in the home including raised toilet seats, chairs with arm rests, removal of throw rugs; use of visual cues and supports for sequential tasks
4	Fine motor control severely compromised, oral motor deficits	Modifications to support participation in self-care tasks, changes in food textures
5	Client severely compromised motorically, dependent with ADLs	Use of environmental controls to allow access to environment

BOX 5-2 Beneficial Approaches for Those with Cognitive Dysfunction

- Use simpler tools for communication than you would use with patients who have do not have cognitive deficits.
- Use simple and more straightforward language and communicate clearly and directly.
- Supervise eating more closely. Patients with frontal lobe abnormalities and poor swallowing ability may have difficulty following medical advice to limit solid foods, or they may place too much food in their mouths.
- Assess the patient's ability to make decisions by talking with him or her and the caretaker, because patients with neurologic disorders are faced with complicated medical, financial, and sometimes legal issues.
- Even those patients with subthreshold cognitive deficits that do not meet criteria for dementia may lack the ability to make sound judgments about their care. Poor insight is very common, so caregiver involvement may be appropriate.
- Supervise walking. Patients with cognitive deficits often have a loss of impulse control and may make poor decisions about where to walk, how far to walk, or when to use equipment such as a walker.
- Remind caregivers and family to try to avoid taking the person's behavior personally.
- Help them understand that there is a physiologic cause for the behavior.
- Encourage the caregiver and family to try to build an atmosphere of comfort and love, with a calm and orderly environment.

Adapted from ALS Association: *ALS, cognitive impairment (CI) and frontotemporal lobar dementia (FTLD): A professional's guide.* Washington, DC, ALS Association, 2005 (alsinfo@alsa-national.org/www.alsa.org).

Spinal Cord Injury

SCI results in quadriplegia or paraplegia. Tetraplegia, referred to as quadriplegia, is any degree of paralysis of the four limbs and trunk musculature. There may be partial upper extremity (UE) function, depending on the level of the cervical lesion. Paraplegia is paralysis of the lower extremities (LEs) with involvement of the trunk and hips, depending on the level of the lesion.

SCIs are referred to in terms of the regions of the spinal cord in which they occur (cervical, thoracic, and lumbar) and the numerical order of the neurologic segments. The level of SCI designates the last fully functioning neurologic segment of the cord. For example, C6 refers to the sixth neurologic segment of the cervical region of the spinal cord as the last fully intact neurologic segment. Complete lesions result in the absence of motor or sensory function of the spinal cord below the level of the injury.

Incomplete lesions may involve several neurologic segments, and some spinal cord function may be partially or completely intact.

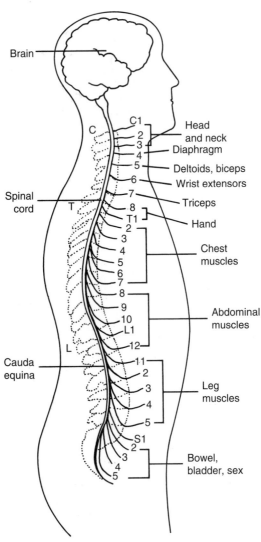

FIGURE 5-4 Spinal nerves and major areas of body they supply. (From Paulson S [ed]: *Santa Clara Valley Medical Center spinal cord injury home care manual,* 2nd ed. San Jose, Calif, Santa Clara Valley Medical Center, 1994.)

The American Spinal Injury Association (ASIA) uses the findings from the neurologic examination to classify injury types to objectify specific clinical findings further:

- ASIA impairment scale classification A indicates a complete lesion; there is no motor or sensory function preserved in the sacral segments S4 through S5. Any preservation of strength without sensory sparing in the sacral segments of S4 through S5 is considered a zone of partial preservation (ZPP) and still considered a complete (ASIA A) neurologic classification.
- ASIA classification B indicates an incomplete lesion in which sensory but not motor function is preserved below the neurologic level; this must include the sacral segments S4 through S5.
- ASIA classification C indicates an incomplete lesion in which motor function is preserved below the neurologic level and more than 50% of the key muscles below the neurologic level have a muscle grade of less than 3 (fair).
- ASIA classification D indicates an incomplete lesion in which motor function is preserved below the neurologic level and at least 50% of the key muscles below the neurologic level have a muscle grade of 3 or more.
- ASIA classification E indicates that motor and sensory functions are normal.

Incomplete injuries are categorized according to the area of damage—central, lateral, anterior, or peripheral.

Central Cord Syndrome

Central cord syndrome occurs when there is more cellular destruction in the center of the cord than in the periphery. Paralysis and sensory loss are greater in the UEs because these nerve tracts are more centrally located than those of the LEs. Central cord syndrome is often seen in older adults in whom arthritic changes have caused a narrowing of the spinal canal; in such cases, cervical hyperextension without vertebral fracture may precipitate central cord damage.

Brown-Sequard Syndrome (Lateral Damage)

Brown-Sequard syndrome results when only one side of the cord is damaged, as in a stabbing or gunshot injury. Below the level of injury, there is motor paralysis and loss of proprioception on the ipsilateral side and loss of pain, temperature, and touch sensation on the contralateral side.

Anterior Spinal Cord Syndrome

Anterior spinal cord syndrome results from injury that damages the anterior spinal artery or the anterior aspect of the cord. This syndrome involves paralysis and loss of pain, temperature, and touch sensation. Proprioception is preserved.

Cauda Equina (Peripheral)

Cauda equina injuries involve peripheral nerves rather than directly involving the spinal cord. This type of injury usually occurs with fractures below the L2 level and results in a flaccid-type paralysis. Because peripheral nerves possess a regenerating capacity that the cord does not, this injury is associated with a better prognosis for recovery. Patterns of sensory and motor deficits are highly variable and asymmetrical.

Conus Medullaris Syndrome

Conus medullaris syndrome involves injury of the sacral cord (conus) and lumbar nerve roots within the neural canal, which usually results in an areflexic bladder, bowel, and LEs.

The following can be used as guidelines to predict and assist the therapist and patients in understanding the recovery process after a new SCI:

- The severity of the original injury determines whether recovery will occur. Unfortunately, no test to measure this severity exists at this time, and predictions must be based on what has happened to others in the past with similar neurologic findings.

- Incomplete injuries are associated with a better chance of further recovery than complete injuries, but even with incomplete injuries there is no guarantee that further recovery will occur.
- Most of the recovery that will occur starts within the first few weeks. Therefore, each day that goes by without any return of function means that the likelihood of recovery is reduced.
- No amount of hard work will cause nerve function to return. If hard work were all it took, very few people would end up with permanent paralysis.
- Rehabilitation will not affect the degree of recovery. The purpose of rehabilitation is to prevent further medical complications through education, maintain and improve the strength and skills that are present, maximize function in self-care activities, facilitate mobility, and optimize lifestyle options for the patient and family, therefore maintaining the body and the individual's general well-being in a recovery ready state.

COMPLICATIONS OF SPINAL CORD INJURY

- Skin breakdown, pressure sores, or decubitus ulcers
- Decreased vital capacity
- Osteoporosis
- Orthostatic hypotension
- Autonomic dysreflexia
- Spasticity
- Heterotopic ossification

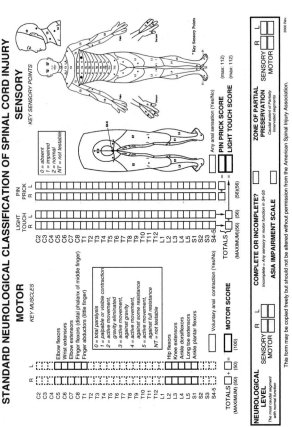

FIGURE 5-5 Standard neurologic classification of spinal cord injury. (Courtesy American Spinal Injury Association, Atlanta, 2000.)

The occupational therapist's general objectives for intervention with the person with SCI are to do the following:

1. Maintain or increase joint ROM and prevent problems associated with body functions and other body structures (skin) via preparatory activities such as active and passive ROM, splinting, positioning, and client education.
2. Increase the strength of all innervated and partially innervated muscles and address problems associated with other body functions (e.g., sensation, higher level cognitive functions, emotional functions) through preparatory activities and engagement in purposeful activities and occupations.
3. Increase physical endurance and other performance skills and performance patterns through engagement in purposeful activities and occupations.
4. Maximize independence in performance in all areas of occupation, including activities of daily living (ADLs), instrumental activities of daily living (IADLs), rest and sleep, education, work, play, leisure, and social participation.
5. Aid in the psychosocial adjustment to disability.
6. Evaluate, recommend, and educate the client in the use and care of necessary durable medical and adaptive equipment.
7. Ensure safe and independent home and environmental accessibility through consultation and safety and accessibility recommendations.
8. Assist the client in developing the communication skills necessary for training caregivers to provide safe assistance.
9. Educate the client and his or her family regarding the benefits and consequences of maintaining healthy and responsible lifestyle habits in relation to long-term function and the aging process.

TABLE 5-10 Expected Functional Outcomes

Level	Functionally Relevant Muscles Innervated	Movement Possible	Patterns of Weakness	NSCISC Sample Size
C1-C3	Sternocleidomastoid: cervical paraspinal; neck accessories	Neck flexion, extension, rotation	Total paralysis of trunk, upper extremities, lower extremities; dependent on ventilator	FIM = 15/ assist = 12
C4	Upper trapezius; diaphragm; cervical paraspinal muscles	Neck flexion, extension, rotation; scapular elevation; inspiration	Paralysis of trunk, upper extremities, lower extremities; inability to cough, endurance and respiratory reserve low secondary to paralysis of intercostals	FIM = 28/ assist = 12
C5	Deltoid, biceps, brachialis, brachioradialis, rhomboids, serratus anterior (partially innervated)	Shoulder flexion, abduction, and extension; elbow flexion and supination; scapular adduction and abduction	Absence of elbow extension, pronation, all wrist and hand movement; total paralysis of trunk and lower extremities	FIM = 36/ assist = 35
C6	Clavicular pectoralis; supinator; extensor carpi radialis longus and brevis; serratus anterior; latissimus dorsi	Scapular protractor; some horizontal adduction, forearm supination, radial wrist extension	Absence of wrist flexion, elbow extension, hand movement; total paralysis of trunk and lower extremities	FIM = 43/ assist = 35
C7-8	Latissimus dorsi; sternal pectoralis; triceps; pronator quadratus; extensor carpi ulnaris; flexor carpi radialis; flexor digitorum profundus and superficialis; extensor communis; pronator/flexor/extensor/abductor pollicis; lumbricals (partially innervated)	Elbow extension; ulnar/wrist extension; wrist flexion; finger flexions and extensions; thumb flexion/extension/abduction	Paralysis of trunk and lower extremities; limited grasp and dexterity secondary to partial intrinsic muscles of the hand	FIM =43/ assist = 35
T1-9	Intrinsics of the hand including thumbs; internal and external intercostals; erector spinae; lumbricals; flexor/extensor/ abductor pollicis	Upper extremities fully intact; limited upper trunk stability; endurance increased secondary to innervation of intercostals	Lower trunk paralysis; total paralysis of lower extremities	FIM =144/ assist =122

				FIM/Assistance Data		
T10-L1	Fully intact intercostals; external obliques; rectus abdominis		Paralysis of lower extremities			FIM =71/ assist =57
L2-S5	Fully intact abdominals and all other trunk muscles; depending on level, some degree of hip flexors, extensor, abductors; knee flexors, extensors; ankle dorsiflexors, plantar flexors	Good trunk stability; partial to full control of lower extremities	Partial paralysis of lower extremities, hips, knees, ankle, foot			FIM =20/ assist =16

	Expected Functional Outcomes	Equipment	Exp	Med	IR
Basic Body Functions					
Level C1-C3					
Respiratory	Ventilator dependent Inability to clear secretions	Two ventilators (bedside, portable) Suction equipment or other suction management device Generator/battery backup			
Bowel	Total assist	Padded reclining shower/commode chair (if roll-in shower available)	1	1	1
Bladder	Total assist		1	1	1
Level C4					
Respiratory	May be able to breathe without a ventilator	If not ventilator free, see C1-C3 for equipment requirements			
Bowel	Total assist	Reclining shower/commode chair (if roll-in shower available)	1	1	1
Bladder	Total assist		1	1	1
Level C5					
Respiratory	Low endurance and vital capacity caused by paralysis of intercostals; may require assist to clear secretions				

Continued

TABLE 5-10 Expected Functional Outcomes—cont'd

	Expected Functional Outcomes	Equipment	FIM/Assistance Data		
			Exp	Med	IR
Bowel	Total assist	Padded shower/commode chair or padded transfer tub bench with commode cutout	1	1	1
Bladder	Total assist	Adaptive devices may be indicated (electric leg bag emptier)	1	1	1
Level C6					
Respiratory	Low endurance and vital capacity secondary to paralysis of intercostals; may require assist to clear secretions				
Bowel	Some total assist	Padded tub bench with commode cutout or padded shower/commode chair Other adaptive devices as indicated	1-2	1	1
Bladder	Some total assist with equipment; may be independent with leg bag emptying	Adaptive devices as indicated	1-2	1	1
Level C7-8					
Respiratory	Low endurance and vital capacity secondary to paralysis of intercostals; may require assist to clear secretions				
Bowel	Some to total assist	Padded tub bench with commode cutout or shower/commode chair Adaptive devices as indicated	1-4	1	1-4
Bladder	Independent to some assist	Adaptive devices as indicated	2-6	3	1-6
Level T1-T9					
Respiratory	Compromised vital capacity and endurance				
Bowel	Independent	Elevated padded toilet seat or padded tub bench with commode cutout	6-7	6	4-6
Bladder	Independent		6	6	5-6

Level T10-L1				
Respiratory	Intact respiratory function			
Bowel	Independent	Padded standard or raised padded toilet seat	6-7	6
Bladder	Independent		6	6
Level L2-S5				
Respiratory	Intact function			
Bowel	Independent	Padded toilet seat	6-7	6
Bladder	Independent		6	6
Mobility, Locomotion, and Safety				
Level C1-C3				
Bed mobility	Total assist	Full electric hospital bed with Trendelenburg feature and side rails	1	1
Bed/wheelchair transfers	Total assist	Transfer board	1	1
		Power or mechanical lift with sling		
Wheelchair propulsion	Manual: total assist	Power recline and/or tilt wheelchair with head, chin, or breath control and manual recliner	6	1-6
	Power: independent with equipment	Vent tray		
Pressure relief/positioning	Total assist; may be independent with equipment	Power recline and/or tilt wheelchair		
		Wheelchair pressure-relief cushion		
		Postural support and head control devices as indicated		
		Hand splints may be indicated		
		Specialty bed or pressure-relief mattress may be indicated		

Continued

TABLE 5-10 Expected Functional Outcomes—cont'd

	Expected Functional Outcomes	Equipment	FIM/Assistance Data		
			Exp	Med	IR
Level C4					
Bed mobility	Total assist	Full electric hospital bed with Trendelenburg feature and side rails			
Bed/wheelchair transfers	Total assist	Transfer board Power or mechanical lift with sling	1	1	1
Wheelchair propulsion	Power: independent Manual: total assist	Power recline and/or tilt wheelchair with head, chin, or breath control and manual recliner Vent tray	6	1	1-6
Pressure relief/ positioning	Total assist; may be independent with equipment	Power recline and/or tilt wheelchair Wheelchair pressure-relief cushion Postural support and head control devices as indicated Hand splints may be indicated Specialty bed or pressure-relief mattress may be indicated			
Level C5					
Bed mobility	Some assist	Full electric hospital bed with Trendelenburg feature with client control Side rails			
Bed/wheelchair transfers	Total assist	Transfer board Power or mechanical lift	1	1	1

Wheelchair propulsion	Power: independent Manual: independent to some assist indoors on noncarpeted, level surface; some to total assist outdoors	Power recline and/or tilt with arm drive control Manual: lightweight rigid or folding frame with handrim modifications	6	6	5-6
Pressure relief/positioning	Independent with equipment	Power recline and/or tilt wheelchair Wheelchair pressure-relief cushion Hand splints Specialty bed or pressure-relief mattress may be indicated Postural support devices		6	
Level C6					
Bed mobility	Some assist	Full electric hospital bed Side rails Full to king standard bed may be indicated		6	
Bed/wheelchair transfers	Level: some assist to independent Uneven: some to total assist	Transfer board Mechanical lift	3	1	1-3
Wheelchair propulsion	Power: independent with standard arm drive on all surfaces Manual: independent indoors; some total assist outdoors	Manual: lightweight rigid or folding frame with modified rims Power: may require power recline or standard upright power wheelchair	6	6	4-6
Pressure relief/positioning	Independent with equipment and/or adapted techniques	Power recline wheelchair Wheelchair pressure-relief cushion Postural support devices Pressure-relief mattress or overlay may be indicated			

Continued

TABLE 5-10 Expected Functional Outcomes—cont'd

	Expected Functional Outcomes	Equipment	FIM/Assistance Data		
			Exp	Med	IR
Level C7-C8					
Bed mobility	Independent to some assist	Full electric hospital bed or full to king standard bed			
Bed/wheelchair transfers	Level: independent Uneven: independent to some assist	With or without transfer board	3-7	4	2-6
Wheelchair propulsion	Manual: independent on all indoor surfaces and level outdoor terrain; some assist with uneven terrain	Manual: rigid or folding lightweight or folding wheelchair with modified rims	6	6	6
Pressure relief/ positioning	Independent	Wheelchair pressure-relief cushion Postural support devices as indicated Pressure-relief mattress or overlay may be indicated			
Level T1-T9					
Bed mobility	Independent	Full to king standard bed			

FIM/assistance data: Exp, expected FIM score; Med, NSCISC median; IR, NSCISC Interquartile Range.

BOX 5-3 Functional Independence Measure Levels

7. Complete independence (timely, safely): No helper
6. Modified independence (device)

Modified Dependence: Helper

5. Supervision
4. Minimal assist (subject = 75% or more)
3. Moderate assist (subject = 50% to 74%)

Complete Dependence

2. Maximal assist (subject = 25%-49%)
1. Total assist (subject = 0%-24%)

Adapted from *Guide for the uniform data set for medical rehabilitation* (including the FIM instrument), Version 5.1. Buffalo, NY, State University of New York at Buffalo, 1997.

Disorders of the Motor Unit

TABLE 5-11	Clinical Manifestations of Peripheral Nerve Lesions of the Brachial Plexus		
Spinal Nerves	**Nerve**	**Motor Distribution**	**Clinical Manifestations**
C5	Dorsal scapular	Rhomboid major and minor, levator scapulae	Loss of scapular elevation, adduction, downward rotation
C5-6	Suprascapular	Supraspinatus, infraspinatus	Weakened lateral rotation of humerus
C5-6	Subscapular	Subscapularis, teres major	Weakened internal rotation of humerus
C5-6	Axillary	Deltoid, teres minor	Loss of shoulder abduction, flexion and external rotation and extension
C5-7	Musculocutaneous	Biceps brachii, brachialis, coracobrachialis	Loss of forearm flexion and supination
C5-7	Long thoracic	Serratus anterior	Winging of the scapula
C6-8	Thoracodorsal	Latissimus dorsi	Loss of arm adduction and shoulder extension
C6-8, T1	Radial	All extensors of arm, wrist, fingers, thumb, abductor pollicis longus, supinator, brachioradialis	Wrist drop, extensor paralysis, inability to supinate
C6-8, T1	Median	Flexors of wrist, hand, and digits; forearm pronators; opponens pollicis; abductor pollicis brevis; flexor pollicis brevis; first and second lumbricales	"Ape-hand" deformity, weakened grip, thenar atrophy, unopposed thumb
C8-T1	Ulnar	Supplies muscles on ulnar side of forearm and hand; adductor pollicis, abductor digiti minimi, opponens digiti minimi, flexor digiti minimi brevis, flexor digitorum profundus (digits 4, 5), third and fourth lumbricales, flexor carpi ulnaris, palmaris brevis, dorsal and palmar interossei, flexor pollicis brevis (deep head)	"Claw-hand" deformity, also known as an intrinsic minus hand deformity, interosseus atrophy, loss of thumb adduction

From Hislop HJ, Montgomery J: *Daniels and Worthingham's muscle testing: techniques of manual examination*, ed 6, Philadelphia, 1995, WB Saunders.

Arthritis

TABLE 5-12 Primary Features of Osteoarthritis and Rheumatoid Arthritis

Feature	Osteoarthritis	Rheumatoid Arthritis
Prevalence	Affects 27 million Americans	Affects 1.3 million Americans
Peak incidence	Increases with age, <50 yr more common in males and >50 yr more common in females	Ages 40-60, 3:1 female-to-male ratio
Onset	Usually develops slowly, over years	Usually develops suddenly, within weeks or months
Systemic features	None	Fever, fatigue, malaise, extraarticular manifestations
Disease process	Noninflammatory, characterized by cartilage destruction	Inflammatory, characterized by synovitis
Joint involvement	Individual	Polyarticular, symmetrical
Joints commonly affected	Neck, spine, hips, knees, MTPs, DIPs, PIPs, thumb CMCs	Neck, jaw, hips, knees, ankles, MTPs, shoulders, elbows, wrists, PIPs, MPs, thumb joints
Morning stiffness	<30 min	At least 1 hr, often >2 hr

CMC, Carpometacarpal; DIP, distal interphalangeal; MTP, metatarsophalangeal; PIP, proximal interphalangeal.

TABLE 5-13 Common Arthritis Medications and Side Effects

Class	Name	Possible Side Effects
Analgesics		
Non-narcotic	Excedrin, Tylenol	Usually none if taken as prescribed
Narcotic	Darvon, Tylenol with codeine, Vicodin	Dizziness or lightheadedness, drowsiness, nausea, vomiting, drug tolerance, and physical dependence with long-term use
Nonsteroidal Anti-Inflammatory Drugs (NSAIDs)		
Traditional	Advil, Aleve, Motrin, Naprosyn	Abdominal pain, dizziness, drowsiness, gastric ulcers and bleeding, greater susceptibility to bruising or bleeding, heartburn, indigestion, lightheadedness, nausea, tinnitus, kidney and liver effects
COX-2 inhibitors	Celebrex	Same as traditional NSAIDs except less likely to cause gastric ulcers and susceptibility to bruising or bleeding; increased risk of heart attack and stroke
Salicylates	Anacin, Bayer, Bufferin	Abdominal cramps, gastric ulcers, increased bleeding tendency, confusion, dizziness, tinnitus, nausea, vomiting, deafness
Corticosteroids	Cortisone, methylprednisone, prednisone	Cushing's syndrome (weight gain, moon face, thin skin, muscle weakness, osteoporosis), cataracts, hypertension, elevated blood sugar, insomnia, mood changes, nervousness or restlessness
Disease-Modifying Antirheumatic Drugs (DMARDs)		
	Gold salts	Sun sensitivity, blood and kidney effects
	Imuran	Immunosuppression
	Methotrexate	Liver and blood effects, decreased fertility
	Penicillamine	Blood and kidney effects
	Plaquenil	Vision damage with long-term use
Biologic Response Modifiers (subset of DMARDs)		
	Enbrel	Headache, injection site irritation
	Humira	Injection site irritation, upper respiratory infection
	Remicade	Infusion reaction, injection site irritation, upper respiratory infection

Evaluation for Arthritis

ONAL THERAPY EVALUATION

It is important to recognize that every client with arthritis has a unique presentation of clinical problems and functional impairment. A strong client-centered and occupation-based approach is helpful in determining each client's specific needs. The evaluation process for clients with arthritis includes many of the same elements as for any physical disability. Special considerations related to arthritis include closer attention to pain, joint stiffness, joint changes or deformity, fatigue, and coping strategies, especially as they relate to activity limitations. Because clients with arthritis typically experience good days and bad days, many symptoms and problems are unpredictable. A thorough systematic assessment of the client's functional, clinical, and psychosocial status is key to prioritizing problems and planning effective intervention.

BOX 5-4 American College of Rheumatology Criteria for Classification of Rheumatoid Arthritis

Stage I: Early
1. No destructive changes on roentgenographic examination*
2. Possible presence of radiographic evidence of osteoporosis

Stage II: Moderate
1. Radiographic evidence of osteoporosis, with or without slight subchondral bone destruction; possible presence of slight cartilage destruction*
2. No joint deformities, although possible limitation of joint mobility*
3. Adjacent muscle atrophy
4. Possible presence of extra-articular soft tissue lesions, such as nodules and tenosynovitis

Stage III: Severe
1. Radiographic evidence of cartilage and bone destruction, in addition to osteoporosis*
2. Joint deformity, such as subluxation, ulnar deviation, or hyperextension, without fibrous or bony ankylosis*
3. Extensive muscle atrophy
4. Possible presence of extra-articular soft tissue lesions, such as nodules and tenosynovitis

Stage IV: Terminal
1. Fibrous or bony ankylosis*
2. Criteria of stage III

*These criteria must be present to permit classification in any particular stage or grade.
From Steinbrocker O, Traeger CH, Batterman RC: Therapeutic criteria in rheumatoid arthritis. *JAMA* 140:659-662, 1949.

TABLE 5-14 Treatment Objectives by Stage of Inflammatory Disease

Stage	Symptoms	Objectives	Treatment Considerations
I. Acute	Pain, inflammation, hot, red joints, tenderness, overall stiffness, limited motion	Decrease pain and inflammation.	Splinting for localized rest day and night, increased bed rest, joint protection, assistive devices, physical agent modalities
		Maintain ROM. Maintain strength and endurance.	Gentle active ROM and/or passive ROM to point of pain (no stretch), proper positioning Functional activities to tolerance, isometric exercises
II. Subacute	Inflammation subsiding, warm, pink joints, decreased pain and tenderness, stiffness limited to morning	Decrease pain and inflammation.	Less restrictive splinting for day, splinting continued at night, joint protection, assistive devices, physical agent modalities
		Maintain ROM. Maintain strength and endurance.	Active ROM and/or passive ROM with gentle stretch, proper positioning Increased functional activities to tolerance, isometric exercises
III. Chronic active	Minimal inflammation, less pain and tenderness, increased activity tolerance, low endurance	Decrease pain and inflammation.	Joint protection, splinting as needed, assistive devices as needed, physical agent modalities as needed
		Increase ROM.	Active ROM and/or passive ROM with stretch at end range
		Increase strength and endurance.	Resistive exercises (isometric or isotonic if no risk of overstressing joints), cardiovascular exercises, increased functional activities
IV. Chronic inactive	No inflammation, pain and stiffness from disuse, low endurance	Decrease pain.	Joint protection, splinting as needed, assistive devices as needed, physical agent modalities as needed
		Increase or maintain ROM.	Active ROM and/or passive ROM with stretch at end range
		Increase strength and endurance.	Resistive exercises (isometric or isotonic if no risk of overstressing joints), cardiovascular exercises, increased functional activities

BOX 5-5   Treatment Precautions Related to Arthritis

- Respect pain.
- Avoid fatigue.
- Avoid placing stress on inflamed or unstable joints.
- Use resistive exercise or activity with caution.
- Be aware of sensory impairments.
- Be cautious with fragile skin caused by systemic disease or pharmacologic side effects.

TABLE 5-15   Splinting Indications by Classification of Progression of Rheumatoid Arthritis

Stage	Symptoms and Radiographic Changes	Splinting Indications
Stage I: Early	No destructive changes, possible osteoporosis	Resting splints to decrease acute inflammation, decrease pain, protect joints
Stage II: Moderate	Osteoporosis with or without slight subchondral bone destruction, slight cartilage destruction, no joint deformities, limited joint mobility possible, muscle atrophy, extraarticular soft tissue lesions possible	Day splints to provide comfort
		Night splints to relieve pain and/or protect joints against potential deformity
		Splints to increase ROM
Stage III: Severe	Cartilage and bone destruction, joint deformity, extensive muscle atrophy, extraarticular soft tissue lesions possible	Day splints to improve function (decrease pain, provide stability, limit undesired motion, properly position joints)
		Night splints to provide positioning and comfort
Stage IV: Terminal	Criteria of stage III, with fibrous and bony ankylosis	Day splints to improve function (decrease pain, provide stability, limit undesired motion, properly position joints)
		Night splints to provide positioning and comfort

BOX 5-6 Principles of Fatigue Management

Attitudes and Emotions

Remove yourself from stressful situations.

Refrain from concentrating on things that make you tense.

Close your eyes, and visualize pleasant places and thoughts.

Body Mechanics

When lifting something that is low, bend your knees and lift by straightening your legs. Try to keep your back straight.

Avoid reaching (use reachers). Avoid stretching, bending, carrying, and climbing. If you have to bend, keep your back straight.

Incorporate good posture into your activities.

Whenever possible, sit when working.

To get up from a chair, slide forward to the edge of the chair. With your feet flat on the floor, lean forward and push with your palms on the arms or seat of the chair. Stand by straightening your legs.

Before you get tired, stop and rest.

Work Pace

Plan on getting 10 to 12 hours of rest daily (naps and at night).

Work at your own pace.

Spread tedious tasks throughout the week.

Do the tasks that require the most energy at the times when you have the most energy.

Alternate easy and difficult activities, and take a 10- to 15-minute rest break each hour.

Leisure Time

Devote a portion of your day to an activity that you enjoy and find relaxing.

Check out what's available in the community.

Work Methods

Keep items within easy reach.

Use good light and proper ventilation and room temperature.

Use joint protection techniques.

Work surfaces should be at a correct height.

Organization

Plan ahead; don't rush or push yourself.

Decide which jobs are absolutely necessary.

Share the workload with family and friends.

How to Begin

Plan ahead by charting your daily routine.

Make a list of tasks, and spread them out in your schedule.

Include daily rest periods and rest breaks during energy-consuming times.

Time	Sun.	Mon.	Tues.	Wed.	Thur.	Fri.	Sat.
7:00 AM							
8:00 AM							
9:00 AM							
10:00 AM							
11:00 AM							
12:00 AM							
1:00 PM							
2:00 PM							
3:00 PM							
4:00 PM							
5:00 PM							
6:00 PM							
7:00 PM							
8:00 PM							
9:00 PM							
10:00 PM							

BOX 5-6   Principles of Fatigue Management—cont'd

Check your schedule for the following factors:
- Is there one day in the week that is longer than the others?
- Are heavier tasks distributed through the week?
- Is there a long task that could be done in several steps?
- Will your plan allow for flexibility?
- Have you devoted part of your day to a relaxing activity?
- Does your plan use the principles of energy conservation?

Hand and Upper Extremity Injuries

TABLE 5-16   Clinical Tests for Specific Dysfunction in the Shoulder

Condition	Pattern of Impairment	Characteristic Findings and Special Tests
Adhesive capsulitis	Loss of active and passive shoulder motion with the most pronounced loss in external rotation and, to a lesser degree, abduction and internal rotation	Capsular end feel to passive motions in restricted planes of movement
Subacromial impingement	Painful arc of motion between ≈ 80 and 100 degrees elevation or at end range of active elevation	In early stages, muscle tests may be strong and painless despite positive impingement test.
Rotator cuff tendinitis	Painful active or resistive rotator cuff muscle use	Painful manual muscle test of scapular plane abduction or external rotation Nonpainful passive motion end ranges Tenderness at tendons of supraspinatus or infraspinatus.
Rotator cuff tear	Significant substitution of scapula with attempted arm elevation	Positive drop arm test Very weak, less than 60% abduction or external rotation

TABLE 5-17 Clinical Tests for Specific Dysfunction in the Wrist

Condition	Pattern of Impairment	Special Tests
Thumb ulnar collateral ligament (gamekeeper's or skier's thumb)	Pain and instability of thumb MP joint	Movement > 35 degrees when valgus instability stress applied to thumb MP joint
Instability of scaphoid	Pain in area of scaphoid bone (anatomic snuffbox) or clunking with movement of wrist	Watson test
		Pain or sound associated with subluxation of dorsal pole of scaphoid while performing test
Instability of distal radioulnar joint	Pain and tenderness in e wrist	Piano keys test
		Hypermobility and pain associated with pressure on distal ulna
Lunate dislocation	Pain or instability in central wrist	Murphy's sign
		Head of third metacarpal level with second and fourth metacarpals while making a fist
Lunotriquetral instability	Pain or instability in central or ulnar wrist	Lunotriquetral ballottement test
		Crepitus; laxity or pain with isolated movement of lunate
TFCC tear	Pain and instability in ulnar wrist	Wrist arthrography or MRI

MRI, Magnetic resonance imaging; TFCC, triangular fibrocartilage complex.

TABLE 5-18 Clinical Tests for Specific Nerve Dysfunction in the Upper Extremity

Condition	Pattern of Impairment	Characteristic Findings and Special Tests
Thoracic outlet syndrome	Nonspecific paresthesias or heaviness with sustained positioning or activity above shoulder level or behind plane of the body	Adson test Roos test
Adverse neural tension	Nonspecific pain or paresthesias with reaching in positions that place tension on brachial plexus nerves	Positive upper limb screening test
Carpal tunnel syndrome	Pain and numbness, primarily in the thumb, index, and middle fingers Usually worse at night; may be associated with activity	Tinel's sign at the wrist Phalen's test Reverse Phalen's test Carpal compression test
Cubital tunnel syndrome	Compression of ulnar nerve at elbow	Elbow fleion test
Ulnar nerve paralysis	Paralysis of adductor pollicis muscle	Froment's, Jeanne's, Wartenberg's sign

TABLE 5-19 Nerve Injuries of the Upper Extremity

Nerve	Location	Affected	Test
Radial nerve (posterior cord, fibers from C5, C6, C7, C8)	Upper arm	Triceps and all distal motors	MMT
		Sensory to SRN	Sensory test
Radial nerve	Above elbow	Brachioradialis and all distal motors	MMT
		Sensory to SRN	Sensory
Radial nerve	At elbow	Supinator, ECRL, ECRB, and all distal motors	MMT
		Sensory to SRN	Sensory
Posterior interosseous nerve	Forearm	ECU, ED, EDM, APL, EPL, EPB, EIP	Wrist extension; if present, indicates PIN rather than high radial nerve
		No sensory	
Radial nerve at ECRB, radial artery, arcade of Frohse, origin of supinator	Radial tunnel syndrome	Weakness of muscles innervated by PIN	Palpate for pain over extensor mass
			Pain with wrist flexion and pronation
		No sensory loss	Pain with wrist extension and supination
			Pain with resisted middle finger extension
Median nerve (lateral from C5, C6, C7; medial cord from C8, T1)	High lesions (elbow and above)	Paralysis/weakness of FCR, PL, all FDS, FDP I and II	MMT
		FPL, pronator teres and quad., opponens pollicis, APB, FPB (radial head), lumbricals I and II	Sensory
		Sensory cutaneous branch of median nerve	
Median nerve	Low (at wrist)	Weakness of thenars only	Inability to flex thumb tip and index fingertip to palm
			Inability to oppose thumb
			Poor dexterity

TABLE 5-19 Nerve Injuries of the Upper Extremity—cont'd

Nerve	Location	Affected	Test
Median nerve under fibrous band in PT, beneath heads of pronator, arch of FDS, origin of FCR	Pronator syndrome	Weakness in thenars, but not muscles innervated by AIN	Provocative tests to isolate compression site
		Sensory in median nerve distribution in hand	
Median nerve under origin of PT, FDS to middle	Anterior interosseous nerve syndrome	Pure motor, no sensory	Inability to flex IP joint of thumb and DIP of index
		Forearm pain precedes paralysis	Increased pain with resisted pronation
		Weakness of FPL, FDP I and II, PQ	Pain with forearm pressure
Median nerve at wrist	Carpal tunnel syndrome	Weakness of medial intrinsics	Provocative tests
		Sensory	Tinel's sign
			Sensory
Ulnar nerve at elbow (branch of medial cord from C7, C8, T1)	Cubital tunnel syndrome	Weakness or paralysis of FCU, FDP III and IV, ulnar intrinsics	Pain with elbow flexion and extension
		Numbness in palmar cutaneous, dorsal cutaneous distribution	
		Loss of grip and pinch strength	
Ulnar nerve at wrist	Compression at canal of Guyon	Weakness and pain in ulnar intrinsics	Reproduced by pressure at site

AIN, Anterior interosseus nerve; APB, abductor pollicis brevis; APL, abductor pollicis longus; ECRB, extensor carpi radialis brevis; ECRL, extensor carpi radialis longus; ECU, extensor carpi ulnaris; ED, extensor digitorum; EDM, extensor digitorum minimus; EIP, extensor indicis proprius; FDS, flexor digitorum superficialis; EPB, extensor pollicis brevis; EPL, extensor pollicis longus; FCR, flexor carpi radialis; FDP, flexor digitorum profundus; FPB, flexor pollicis brevis; FPL, flexor pollicis longus; MMT, manual muscle test; PIN, posterior interosseous nerve; PQ, pronator quadratus; PT, pronator teres; SRN, superficial radial nerve.

Hip Fractures and Lower Extremity Joint Replacement

The older adult population is most at risk for hip fractures. Reduced mobility and the presence of osteoporosis are two specific risk factors. Older women, in particular, develop osteoporosis to a greater degree than men and thus tend to have more hip fractures when they fall.

BOX 5-7 Weight-Bearing Restrictions

NWB (non–weight bearing) indicates that no weight at all can be placed on the extremity involved.

TTWB (toe-touch weight bearing) indicates that only the toe can be placed on the ground to provide some balance while standing—90% of the weight is still on the unaffected leg. In toe-touch weight bearing, clients are instructed to imagine that an egg is under their foot.

PWB (partial weight bearing) indicates that only 50% of the person's body weight can be placed on the affected leg.

WBAT (weight bearing at tolerance) indicates that clients are allowed to judge how much weight they are able to put on the affected leg without causing too much pain.

FWB (full weight bearing) indicates that clients should be able to put 100% of their weight on the affected leg without causing damage to the fracture site.

From Early MB: *Physical dysfunction: Practical skills for the occupational therapy assistant.* St. Louis, Mosby, 1998.

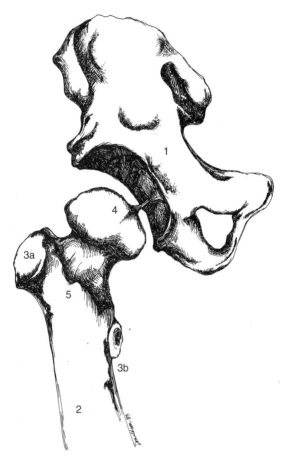

FIGURE 5-6 Normal hip anatomy. 1, Acetabulum. 2, Femur. 3a, Greater trochanter. 3b, Lesser trochanter. 4, Ligamentum teres. 5, Intertrochanteric crest. (Adapted from Croch JE: *Functional human anatomy,* 3rd ed. Philadelphia, Lea & Febiger, 1978; and Grant LC: *Grant's atlas of anatomy,* 6th ed. Baltimore, Williams & Wilkins, 1972.)

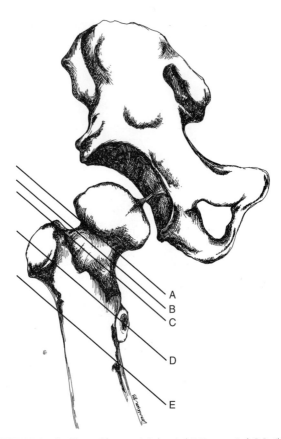

FIGURE 5-7 Levels of femoral fracture. **A,** Subcapital. **B,** Transcervical. **C,** Basilar. **D,** Intertrochanteric. **E,** Subtrochanteric. (Adapted from Crow I: Fractures of the hip: A self study. *ONA J* 5:12-32, 1978.)

BOX 5-8 Hip Precautions

Posterolateral Approach
- No hip flexion greater than 90 degrees
- No internal rotation
- No adduction (crossing legs or feet)

Anterolateral Approach
- No external rotation
- No adduction (crossing legs or feet)
- No extension

From Early MB: *Physical dysfunction: Practical skills for the occupational therapy assistant.* St. Louis, Mosby, 1998.

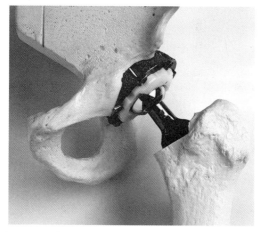

FIGURE 5-8 Hip prothesis. (From Black J, Hawks J: *Medical-surgical nursing: Clinical management for positive outcomes,* 8th ed. St. Louis, Elsevier, 2009.)

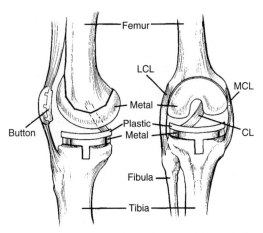

FIGURE 5-9 Total knee replacement. The metal aspects of the prosthesis cover the distal portion of the femur and the end of the tibia. There is a polyethylene plastic–bearing surface (plastic) between the metallic aspects of the two surfaces. The patella is replaced by a polyethylene button. The medial collateral ligament (MCL), lateral collateral ligament (LCL), and cruciate ligaments (CL) are retained. (Adapted from Early MB: Physical dysfunction: *Practical skills for the occupational therapy assistant.* St. Louis, Mosby, 1998.)

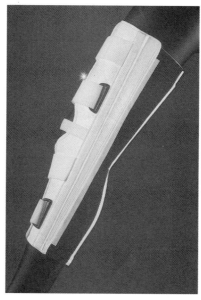

FIGURE 5-10 A knee immobilizer is used to support and stabilize the knee joint during mobility. (From Ignatavicius D, Workman ML: *Medical-surgical Nursing: Patient-centered collaborative care,* 6th ed. St. Louis, Elsevier, 2010.)

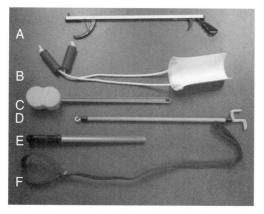

FIGURE 5-11 Assistive devices for ADLs. *Top to bottom,* Reacher, sock aid, long-handled sponge, dressing stick, long-handled shoe horn, and leg lifter.

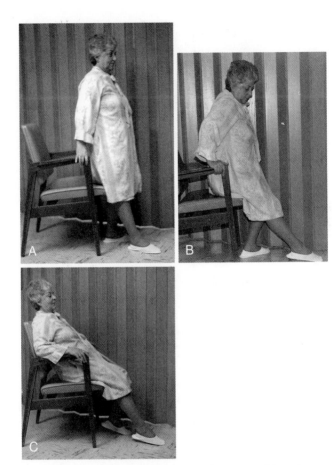

FIGURE 5-12 Chair transfer technique. **A,** Client extends operated leg and reaches for arm rests. **B, C,** Bearing some weight on the arms, the client sits down slowly, maintaining some extension of the operated leg.

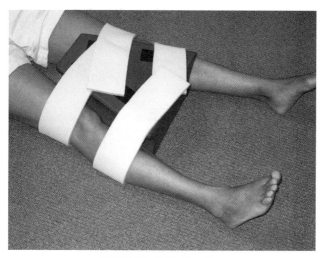

FIGURE 5-13 Abduction wedge.

Training Procedures for Persons with Hip Surgery

- Bed mobility
- Transfers
  - Chair
  - Commode chair
  - Shower stall
  - Shower over tub (without shower doors)
  - Car
- Lower body dressing
- Lower body bathing
- Hair shampoo
- Homemaking
- Caregiver training

Training Procedures for Persons with Total Knee Replacement

- Bed mobility
- Transfers
- Lower extremity dressing

SPECIAL EQUIPMENT

The occupational therapist (OT) should be familiar with the following equipment, which is commonly used in the treatment of hip fractures and total hip replacement.

Hemovac

During surgery, a plastic drainage tube is inserted at the surgical site to assist with postoperative drainage of blood. It has an area for collection of drainage and may be connected to a portable suction machine. The unit should not be disconnected for any activity because this may create a blockage in the system. The Hemovac is usually left in place for 2 days after surgery.

Abduction Wedge

Large and small triangular foam wedges (Fig. 5-13) are used when the client is supine to maintain the LEs in the abducted position.

Balanced Suspension

This is fabricated and set up by an orthopedic technician and can be used for approximately 3 days after surgery. It balances the weight of the elevated leg by weights placed at the opposite end of the pulley system. Its purpose is to support the affected LE in the first few postoperative days. The client's leg can be taken out of the device for exercise only.

Reclining Wheelchair

A wheelchair with an adjustable back rest that allows a reclining position is used for clients who have hip flexion precautions while sitting.

Commode Chairs

The use of a commode chair instead of the regular toilet aids in safe transfers and allows the client to observe necessary hip flexion precautions.

Sequential Compression Devices

Sequential compression devices (SCDs) are used postoperatively to reduce the risk of deep vein thrombosis (DVT). They are inflatable external leggings that provide intermittent pneumatic compression of the legs.

Antiembolus Hose

These are thigh-high hosiery that are worn 24 hours/day and removed only during bathing. Their purpose is to assist circulation, prevent edema, and thus reduce the risk of DVT.

Patient-Controlled Analgesia

Patient-controlled analgesia (PCA) is analgesia delivered through an IV line and controlled by the patient; PCEA is patient-controlled epidural analgesia delivered through an epidural line. A prescribed amount of medication is programmed by the physician and nursing staff to allow the client to self-administer pain medication by pushing a button to inject a safe amount. When dosages have reached a limit, the machine will not administer medication, even if the button is pushed.

Incentive Spirometer

This portable breathing apparatus is used to encourage deep breathing and prevent the development of postoperative pneumonia.

Continuous Passive Motion Machine

Continuous passive motion (CPM) machine is a mechanical device that supports a joint and can be set to move slowly through a designated ROM to promote controlled movement in the operated joint.

Low Back Pain

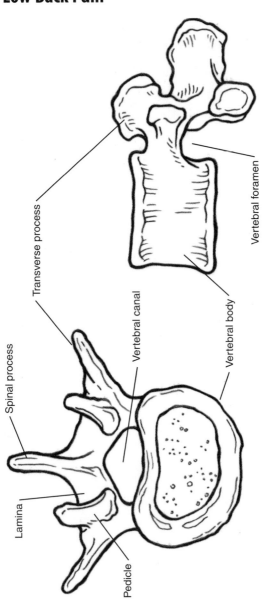

FIGURE 5-14 Vertebrae from above and side view.

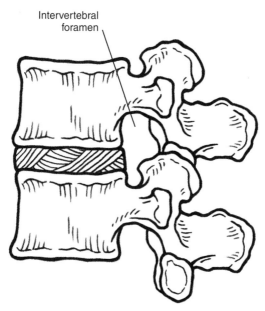

FIGURE 5-15 Two vertebrae in articulation. The spinal nerve exits via the intervertebral foramen.

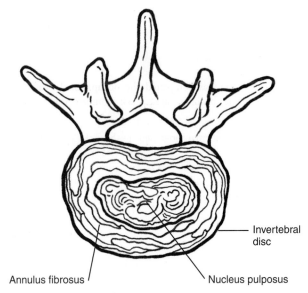

FIGURE 5-16 Cut surface of the disc.

Occupational Therapy Interventions for Low Back Pain

On the basis of the client's evaluation, the therapist develops an intervention plan that may use any or all of the following:

- Education regarding normal back anatomy and the physiology of back movement as they relate to performance of occupations
- Use of neutral spine back stabilization in occupational performance to reduce pain
- Education in basic body mechanics
- Training in use of adaptive equipment to modify tasks
- Task analysis and use of ergonomic design to modify the environment
- Training in use of energy conservation to maintain participation in occupation

- Use of occupation to increase strength and endurance
- Education in strategies for pain management, stress reduction, and coping
- Analysis of occupation

After the client has completed the occupational profile and identified specific problem areas, ask yourself the following questions:

- What is the normal movement in this activity? Analyze the activity.
- What separate movements make up this activity?
- Which movements could trigger pain in this client?

Now, plan for how this intervention will be provided:

- How can this activity be performed properly to avoid the position that causes pain?
- Could the environment be changed or adapted?

Burns and Burn Rehabilitation

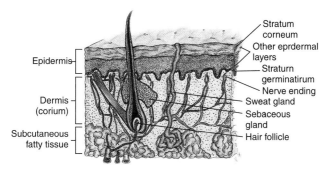

FIGURE 5-17 Cross section of skin. (From Potter PA, Perry AG: *Fundamentals of nursing,* 7th ed. St. Louis, Elsevier, 2009.)

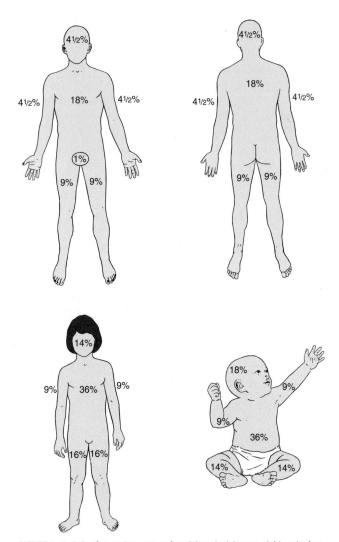

FIGURE 5-18 Rule of nines. Proportions for adult and adolescent, child, and infant. Note the relatively greater surface area of the head and slightly lesser surface area of the lower extremities in young children when compared with adults. (From Mosby: *Mosby's Dictionary of medicine, nursing, & health professions,* 7th ed. St. Louis, Elsevier, 2009.)

Modified Lund and Browder Chart						% Partial-thickness	% Full-thickness	% Total
Area	Age (Years)							
	0-1	1-4	5-9	10-15	Adult			
Head	19	17	13	10	7			
Neck	2	2	2	2	2			
Ant. trunk	13	13	13	13	13			
Post. trunk	13	13	13	13	13			
R. buttock	2.5	2.5	2.5	2.5	2.5			
L. buttock	2.5	2.5	2.5	2.5	2.5			
Genitalia	1	1	1	1	1			
R. U. arm	4	4	4	4	4			
L. U. arm	4	4	4	4	4			
R. L. arm	3	3	3	3	3			
L. L. arm	3	3	3	3	3			
R. hand	2.5	2.5	2.5	2.5	2.5			
L. hand	2.5	2.5	2.5	2.5	2.5			
R. thigh	5.5	6.5	8.5	8.5	9.5			
L. thigh	5.5	6.5	8.5	8.5	9.5			
R. leg	5	5	5.5	6	7			
L. leg	5	5	5.5	6	7			
R. foot	3.5	3.5	3.5	3.5	3.5			
L. foot	3.5	3.5	3.5	3.5	3.5			
					Total			

FIGURE 5-19 Modified Lund and Browder chart. Burn size can be determined most accurately in children by using this chart, which accounts for changes in the size of body parts that occur with growth. (Adapted from Lund CC, Browder NC: The estimation of areas of burns. *Surg Gynecol Obstet* 79:352, 1944.)

TABLE 5-20 Burn Wound Characteristics

Burn Depth	Common Causes	Tissue Depth	Clinical Findings	Healing Time	Scar Potential
Superficial (first degree)	Sunburn, brief flash burns, brief exposure to hot liquids or chemicals	Superficial epidermis	Erythema, dry, no blisters, short-term moderate pain	3-7 days	No potential for hypertrophic scar or contractures
Superficial partial thickness (superficial second degree) and donor sites	Severe sunburn or radiation burns, prolonged exposure to hot liquids, brief contact with hot metal objects	Epidermis, upper dermis	Erythema, wet, blisters; significant pain	<2 wk	Minimal potential for hypertrophy or contractures if healing not delayed by secondary infection or further trauma
Deep partial thickness (deep second degree)	Flames; firm or prolonged contact with hot metal objects; prolonged contact with hot, viscous liquids	Epidermis and much of dermis nonviable, but survival of skin appendages from which skin may regenerate	Erythema; larger, usually broken blisters on skin with hair; on glabrous skin of palms and soles of feet, large, possibly intact blisters over beefy red dermis; severe pain to even light touch	>2 wk; may convert to full thickness with onset of infection	High potential for hypertrophic scarring and contractures across joints, web spaces, and facial contours; high risk for boutonnière deformities if dorsal fingers involved

Full thickness (third degree)	Extreme heat or prolonged exposure to heat, hot objects, or chemicals for extended periods	Epidermis and dermis: nonviable skin appendages and nerve endings	Pale, nonblanching, dry, coagulated capillaries possible; no sensation to light touch except at deep partial-thickness borders	Surgical intervention required for wound closure in larger areas; possible for smaller areas to heal in from borders over extended period of time	Extremely high potential for hypertrophic scarring or contractures, depending on method used for wound closure
Subdermal	Electrical burns and severe long-duration burns (e.g., house fires, entrapment in or under a burning motor vehicle or hot exhaust system, smoking in bed or alcohol-related burns)	Full-thickness burn with damage to underlying tissue	Possible charring of nonviable surface, or, with exposed fat, possible presence of small external wounds on tendons, muscles; with electrical injuries, possibility for small external wounds with significant secondary subdermal tissue loss and peripheral nerve damage	Requires surgical intervention for wound closure; may require amputation or significant reconstruction	Similar to full-thickness burns except when amputation removes burn site

TABLE 5-21 Burn Rehabilitation Evaluation Components

Initial Evaluation	Inpatient Rehabilitation	Outpatient Rehabilitation
Burn cause	Graft adherence	
%TBSA, depth of burn	Skin or scar condition	Skin or scar condition
Area(s) involved	Contracture concerns	Compression garment fit
Age, hand dominance	Edema (if present)	Volumetrics if needed
Functional status	ADL performance level	ADL performance level
Occupation	Work skills	Work skills
ROM and strength	Active and passive ROM, TAM	Active and passive ROM, TAM
Mobility and activity tolerance	Strength and activity tolerance	Strength and activity tolerance
Developmental level (child)	Developmental level (child)	Developmental level (child)
Psychological status	Psychological status	Psychological status
Social support	Social support	Social support
Leisure activities	Leisure activities Compression garment needs Home management	Leisure activities Compression garment needs Home management Home care understanding Return to work capacity Return to school potential and need for reentry program

ADLs, Activities of daily living; ROM, range of motion; TAM, total active motion; TBSA, total body surface area.

TABLE 5-22 Antideformity Positioning for Specific Body Areas Following Burn Injury

Body Area	Antideformity Position	Equipment and Technique
Neck	Neutral to slight extension	No pillow; soft collar, neck conformer, or triple-component neck splint
Chest and abdomen	Trunk extension, shoulder retraction	Lower top of bed, towel roll beneath thoracic spine, clavicle straps
Axilla	Shoulder abduction 90-100 degrees	Arm boards, airplane splint, clavicle straps, overhead traction
Elbow and forearm	Elbow extension, forearm neutral	Pillows, armboards, conformer splints, dynamic splints
Wrist and hand	Wrist extension 30 degrees, thumb abducted and extended, MP flexion 50-70 degrees, IP extension	Elevate with pillows, volar burn hand splint
Hip and thigh	Neutral extension, hips 10-15 degrees abduction	Trochanter rolls, pillow between knees, wedges
Knee and lower leg	Knee extension; anterior burn: slight flexion	Knee conformer, casts, elevation when sitting, dynamic splints
Ankle and foot	Neutral to 0-5 degrees dorsiflexion	Custom splint, cast, AFO
Ears and face	Prevent pressure	No pillows; headgear

AFO, Ankle-foot orthosis; IP, Interphalangeal; MP, Metacarpophalangeal.

Amputation and Prosthetic

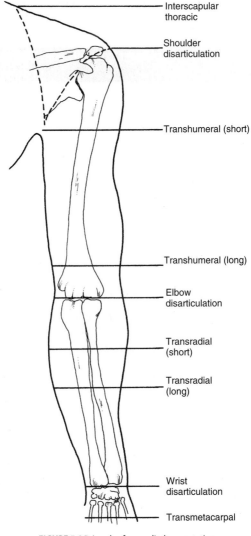

FIGURE 5-20 Levels of upper limb amputation.

Sensation

- Neuroma
- Phantom limb
- Phantom sensation

Component Parts of the Upper Extremity Body-Powered Prosthesis

- Prosthetic sock
- Socket
- Harness and control system
- Terminal device
- Wrist unit

TABLE 5-23 Amputation Levels, Functional Losses, and Suggested Prosthetic Components

Level of Amputation	Loss of Function	Suggested Functional Prosthetic Components
Partial hand	Some or all grip functions	Dependent on cosmesis and functional loss
Wrist disarticulation	Hand and wrist function; ≈ 50% of pronation and supination	Harness, control cable, socket, flexible elbow hinges
Long transradial	Hand and wrist function; most pronation and supination	Same as for wrist disarticulation but circular wrist unit
Short transradial	Hand and wrist function; all pronation and supination; half cuff, wrist unit, and terminal device	Harness, control cable, self-suspending socket or traditional socket with rigid elbow hinge, wrist unit and terminal device extension
Elbow disarticulation	Hand and wrist function; all pronation and supination; elbow flexion and extension	Harness, dual-control cables, socket, externally locking elbow, forearm shell, wrist unit, and terminal device
Long transhumeral	Hand and wrist function; all pronation and supination; most shoulder internal and external rotation elbow flexion and extension	Harness, dual-control cables, socket, internally locking elbow, lift assist, turntable, forearm shell, wrist unit, and terminal device
Short transhumeral	All of the above; shoulder internal and external rotation	Same as for long transhumeral, but socket may partially cover shoulder, restricting its function
Shoulder disarticulation	Loss of all arm and hand functions	Same as for long transhumeral, but socket covers much of the chest wall shoulder; chest strap; shoulder unit; upper arm shell; chin-operated nudge control for elbow unit
Interscapular thoracic	Loss of all arm and hand functions; partial or complete loss of clavicle and scapula	May be same as above but with lightweight materials; when minimal function is attainable, endoskeletal cosmetic prosthesis sometimes preferred
Bilateral amputation	Dependent on levels of amputation	Appropriate to level of amputation, plus wrist flexion unit and cable-operated wrist rotator

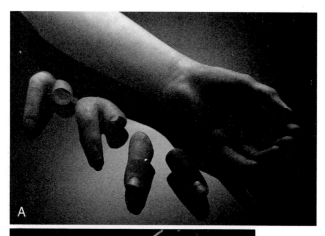

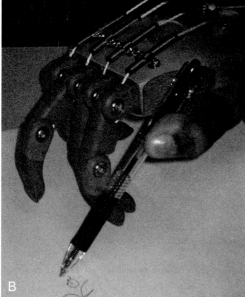

FIGURE 5-21 Prostheses for a partial hand amputation. (**A,** Courtesy Otto Bock HealthCare, Minneapolis; **B,** courtesy Touch Bionics, Hilliard Ohio, 2009.)

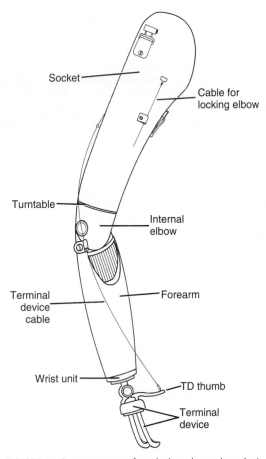

FIGURE 5-22 Component parts of standard transhumeral prosthesis.

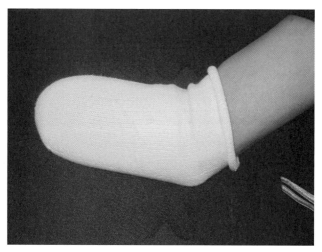

FIGURE 5-23 Prosthetic sock worn under the prosthesis.

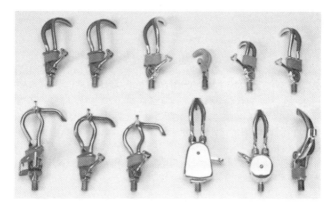

FIGURE 5-24 The Hosmer-Dorrance hook terminal devices are available in a variety of materials, shapes, and sizes that can be matched to the particular functional needs of a child or adult. (Courtesy Hosmer-Dorrance, Campbell, Calif.)

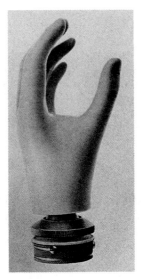

FIGURE 5-25 Ball-and-socket wrist unit. (Courtesy Otto Bock HealthCare, Minneapolis.)

BOX 5-9   Interventions for Body Functions, Body Structures, and Performance Skills

- Improve body image, self-image, psychosocial adjustment.
- Promote independent function during ADLs and IADLs.
- Promote wound healing.
- Improve desensitization of the limb.
- Establish pain management practices.
- Promote residual limb shaping and shrinking.
- Promote proper skin hygiene.
- Promote care of insensate skin.
- Maintain and restore passive and active range of motion.
- Maintain and restore upper body strength and endurance.
- Improve understanding of prosthetic components and options.
- Recommend appropriate prosthetic components.

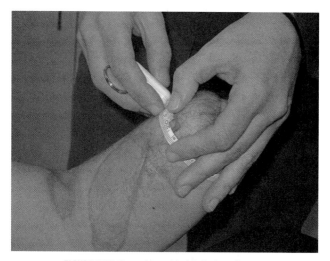

FIGURE 5-26 Measuring residual limb circumference.

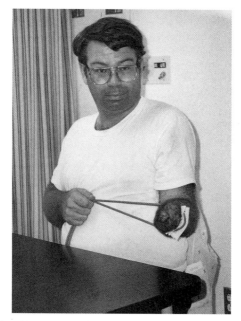

FIGURE 5-27 Home program of upper limb strengthening to prepare arm for prosthesis. Resistance tubing is being used for resistive exercise.

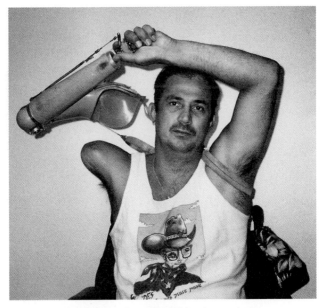

FIGURE 5-28 Coat method of donning prosthesis.

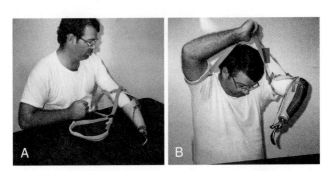

FIGURE 5-29 Sweater method of donning prosthesis.

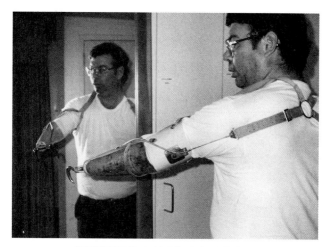

FIGURE 5-30 Control training in front of mirror.

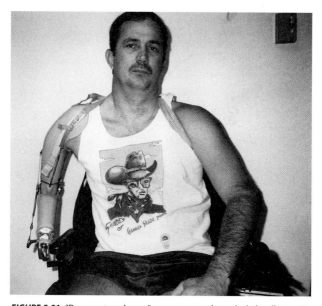

FIGURE 5-31 "Down, out, and away" movement used to unlock the elbow unit.

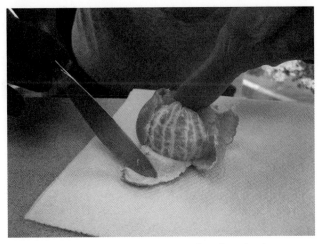

FIGURE 5-32 Prehension training with an electric hand.

BOX 5-10 Advantages and Disadvantages of a Myoelectric Prosthesis

Advantages
1. Improved cosmesis
2. Increased grip force (approximately 25 lb in an adult myoelectric hand)
3. Minimal or no harnessing
4. Ability to use overhead
5. Minimal effort needed to control
6. Control more closely corresponding to human physiologic control

Disadvantages
1. Cost of prosthesis
2. Frequency of maintenance and repair
3. Fragile nature of glove and necessity of frequent replacements
4. Lack of sensory feedback (a body-powered prosthesis has some sense of proprioceptive feedback)
5. Slowness in responsiveness of electric hand
6. Increased weight

Hybrid Prostheses

- Identification of potential muscle sites
- Muscle site control training

Prosthetic Program

- Orientation and education
- Control training
- Use training
- Functional training

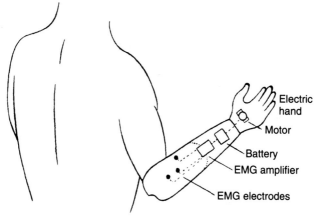

FIGURE 5-33 Electric-powered myoelectrically controlled, transradial prosthesis with an electromechanical hand terminal device activated by electromyographic potentials. (From Billock JN: Upper limb prosthetic terminal devices: Hands versus hooks. *Clin Prosthet Orthot* 10:57-65, 1986.)

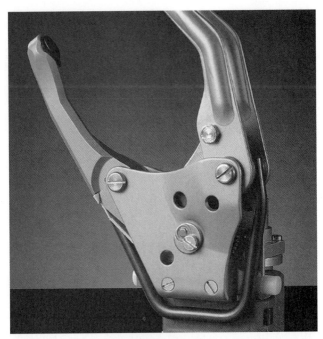

FIGURE 5-34 The Sensor HandSpeed. (Courtesy Otto Bock HealthCare, Minneapolis.)

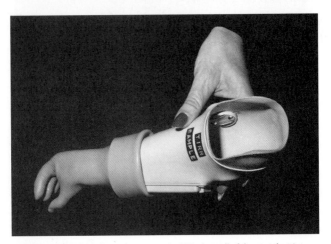

FIGURE 5-35 Surface electrodes, recessed within the wall of the myoelectric socket, detect muscle contractions.

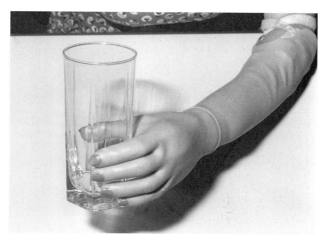

FIGURE 5-36 When approaching the glass, the hand is prepositioned in midline to grasp the glass as a normal hand.

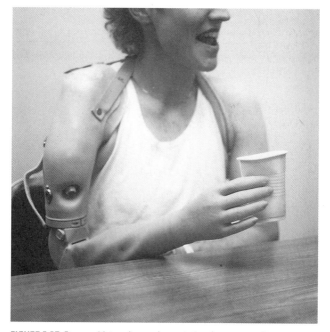

FIGURE 5-37 Person with transhumeral amputation demonstrates how excessive grasp crushes the object (plastic cup) being held.

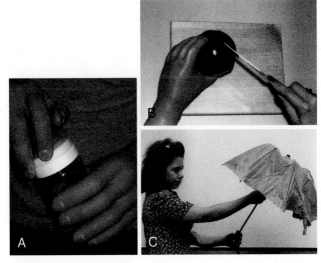

FIGURE 5-38 Activities of daily living. **A,** Opening a jar is accomplished with the myoelectric hand holding the jar and the sound hand turning the lid. **B,** Cutting an apple is accomplished with the myoelectric hand holding the apple while the sound hand holds the knife to cut. **C,** Opening an umbrella is accomplished by holding the base knob of the umbrella with the myoelectric hand and using the sound hand to open as normal.

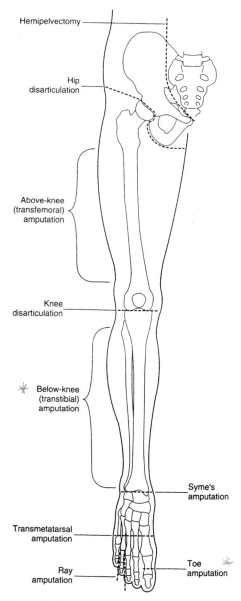

FIGURE 5-39 Levels of lower extremity amputation. (From Paz JC, West MP: *Acute care handbook for physical therapists,* 2nd ed. Oxford, England, Butterworth-Heinemann, 2002.)

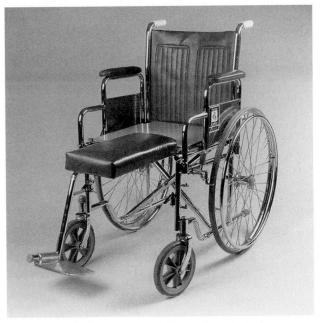

FIGURE 5-40 Wheelchair with support for residual limb.

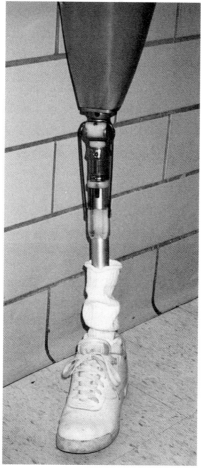

FIGURE 5-41 Typical pylon.

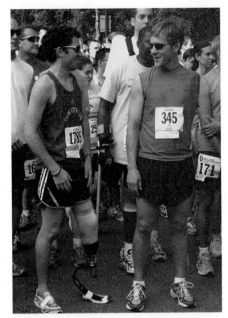

FIGURE 5-42 Athlete with a specialized running prosthesis at the start of a race. (From Chalufour M: Reasons to run: Unexpected perspectives. *Running Times* 330:35, 2005.)

Cardiac and Pulmonary Disease

The heart and blood vessels work together to maintain a constant flow of blood throughout the body. The heart, located between the lungs, is pear-shaped and about the size of a fist. It functions as a two-sided pump. The right side pumps blood from the body to the lungs; the left side simultaneously pumps blood from the lungs to the body. Each side of the heart has two chambers, an upper atrium and a lower ventricle.

Blood flows to the heart from the venous system. The blood enters the right atrium, which contracts and squeezes the blood into the right ventricle. Next, the right ventricle contracts and ejects the blood into the lungs, where carbon dioxide is exchanged for oxygen. Oxygen-rich blood flows from the lungs to the left atrium. As the left atrium contracts, it forces blood into the left ventricle, which then contracts and ejects its contents into the aorta for systemic circulation (Fig. 5-43). Blood travels from the aorta to the arteries and through progressively smaller blood vessels to networks of very tiny capillaries. In the capillaries, blood cells exchange their oxygen for carbon dioxide.

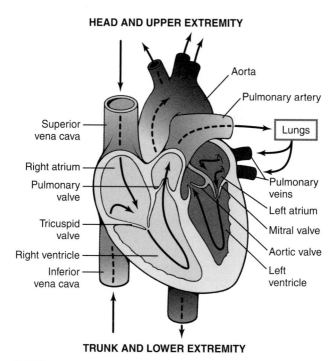

FIGURE 5-43 Anatomy of the heart. (From Thibodeau GA, Patton KT: *The human body in health and disease,* 5th ed . St. Louis, Elsevier, 2010.)

Each of the ventricles has two valves, an input valve and an output valve. The valves open and close as the heart muscle (myocardium) contracts and relaxes. These valves control the direction and flow of blood. The input valves are the mitral, or bicuspid, valve (between the left atrium and ventricle) and the tricuspid valve (between the right atrium and ventricle). The output valves are the aortic and pulmonary valves.

The heart is living tissue and requires a blood supply through an arterial and venous system of its own, or it will die. Coronary arteries cross over the myocardium to supply it with oxygen-rich blood. The coronary arteries are named for their location on the myocardium (Fig. 5-44). Cardiologists generally refer to these arteries by

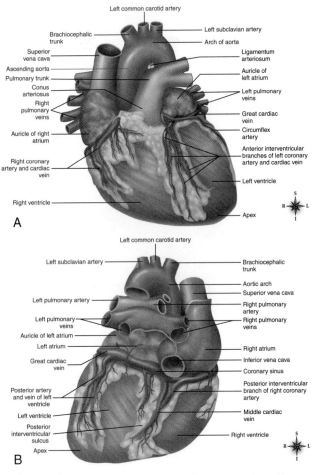

FIGURE 5-44 Coronary circulation. (From Andreoli TE, Benjamin IJ, Griggs RC, Wing EJ: *Andreoli and carpenter's cecil essentials of medicine,* 8th ed. Philadelphia, Elsevier, 2010.)

abbreviations, such as LAD for the left anterior descending and RCA for the right coronary artery. The LAD is on the left anterior portion of the heart and runs in a downward direction, supplying part of the left ventricle. A blockage of this coronary artery will interrupt the blood supply to the left ventricle. Because the left ventricle supplies the body and brain with blood, a heart attack caused by LAD blockage can have serious consequences.

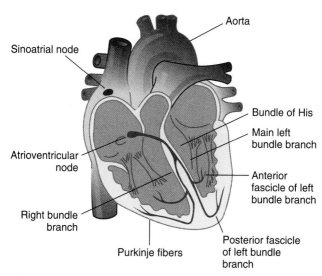

FIGURE 5-45 Cardiac conduction. (From Hall JE, Guyton AC: *Guyton and Hall textbook of medical physiology,* 12th ed. Philadelphia, Elsevier, 2011.)

TABLE 5-24 Comparison of Three Methods of Assessing Cardiovascular Disability

	Method		
Class	New York Heart Association Functional Classification	Canadian Cardiovascular Society Functional Classification	Specific Activity Scale
I	Patients with cardiac disease but without resulting limitations of physical activity; ordinary physical activity does not cause undue fatigue, palpitation, dyspnea, or anginal pain.	Ordinary physical activity, such as walking and climbing stairs, does not cause angina; angina with strenuous or rapid prolonged exertion at work or recreation.	Patients can perform to completion any activity requiring ≥7 metabolic equivalents (METs)—e.g., can carry 24 lb up eight steps; do outdoor work [shovel snow, spade soil]; do recreational activities [skiing, basketball, squash, handball], jog or walk 5 mph
II	Patients with cardiac disease resulting in slight limitation of physical activity; comfortable at rest; ordinary physical activity results in fatigue, palpitation, dyspnea, or anginal pain.	Slight limitation of ordinary activity; walking or climbing stairs rapidly, walking uphill, walking or stair climbing after meals, in cold, in wind, or when under emotional stress, or only during the few hours after awakening; walking more than two blocks on the level and climbing more than one flight of ordinary stairs at a normal pace and in normal conditions.	Patients can perform to completion any activity requiring ≤5 METs)—e.g., have sexual intercourse without stopping, garden, rake, weed, roller skate, dance fox trot, walk at 4 mph on level ground, but cannot and do not perform to completion activities requiring ≥ 7 METs
III	Patients with cardiac disease resulting in marked limitation of physical activity; comfortable at rest; less than ordinary physical activity causes fatigue, palpitation, dyspnea, or anginal pain.	Marked limitation of ordinary physical activity; walking one to two blocks on the level and climbing one flight in normal conditions.	Patients can perform to completion any activity requiring ≤2 METs—e.g., shower without stopping, strip and make bed, clean windows, walk 2.5 mph, bowl, play golf, dress without stopping, but cannot and do not perform to completion any activities requiring > 5 METs
IV	Patient with cardiac disease resulting in inability to carry on any physical activity without discomfort; symptoms of cardiac insufficiency or of anginal syndrome may be present, even at rest; if any physical activity is undertaken, discomfort is increased.	Inability to carry on any physical activity without discomfort; anginal syndrome may be present at rest.	Patients cannot or do not perform to completion activities requiring >2 METs; cannot carry out activities listed above (specific activity scale III)

Adapted from Goldman L, Hashimoto B, Cook EF, Loscalzo A: Comparative reproducibility and validity of systems for assessing cardiovascular functional class: Advantages of a new specific activity scale. *Circulation* 64:1227–1234, 1981; and from UpToDate: Comparison of Three Methods Of Assessing Cardiovascular Disability, 2012 (http://www.uptodate.com/contents/image?imageKey=CARD/1346).

TABLE 5-25 Common Cardiac Medications

Category	Name of Medication (Generic and Trade Name)	Purpose and Uses	Reason Prescribed
Angiotensin II receptor blockers (or inhibitors)	Losartan (Cozaar) Irbesartan (Avopro)	Keep blood pressure from rising by preventing angiotensin II from having an effect on heart	Control high blood pressure. Control heart failure.
Beta blockers	Atenolol (Tenormin) Propranolol (Inderal)	Decrease heart rate and cardiac output, lowering blood pressure and making heart beat more slowly and with less force	Treat of abnormal cardiac rhythms and chest pain.
Calcium channel blockers	Amlodipine (Norvasc, Letrel) Diltiazem (Cardizem, Tiazac)	Interrupt movement of calcium into cells of heart and blood vessels	Treat high blood pressure, angina, and some arrhythmias.
Diuretics (water pills)	Furosemide (Lasis) Hydroclorothiazide (EsiDrix, Hydrodiuril)	Cause loss of excess water and sodium by urination	Lower blood pressure. Reduce edema in lungs and extremities.
Vasodilators	Nitroglycerin Minoxidil	Relax blood vessels Increase supply of blood and oxygent to the heart while reducing its workload	Ease chest pain.
Digitalis preparations	Digoxin Lanoxin	Increase force of cardiac contractions	Treat heart failure, arrythmias, and atrial fibrilation.
Statins	Statins Resins Nicotinic acid (Niacin)	Lower blood cholosterol levels	Lower LDL, raise HDL, and lower triglyceride levels.
Anticoagulants	Warfarin (Coumadin)	Decrease blood-clotting time	Prevent clots from forming. Prevent strokes.
Antiplatelet agents	Aspirine Dipyridamole	Prevent clots by preventing platelets from sticking together	Prevent clots after MI and with unstable angina, ischemic stroke, and plaque.
ACE inhibitors	Fosinopril (Monopril)	Expand blood vessels, lower levels of angiotensin II Make heart work more easily	Treat high blood pressure and heart failure.

ACE, Angiotensin-converting enzyme; HDL, high-density lipoprotein; LDL, low-density lipoprotein; MI, myocardial infarction.

TABLE 5-26 Signs and Symptoms of Cardiac Distress

Sign or Symptom	What to Look For
Angina	Chest pain that may be described as squeezing, tightness, aching, burning, or choking. Pain is generally substernal and may radiate to the arms, jaw, neck, or back. More intense or longer lasting pain forewarns of greater ischemia.
Dyspnea	Shortness of breath with activity or at rest. Note the activity that brought on the dyspnea and the amount of time that it takes to resolve. Dyspnea at rest, and with resting respiratory rate >r 30 breaths/min, are signs of acute CHF. The patient may require emergency medical help.
Orthopnea	Dyspnea brought on by lying supine. Count the number of pillows that the patient needs to breathe comfortably during sleep (one to four pillows needed to relieve orthopnea).
Nausea/emesis	Vomiting or signs that the patient feels sick to the stomach
Diaphoresis Fatigue	Cold, clammy sweat, generalized feeling of exhaustion. The Borg rate of perceived exertion (RPE) scale is a tool used to grade fatigue (see Box 5-11).
Cerebral signs	Ataxia, dizziness, confusion, and fainting (syncope) are all signs that the brain is not getting enough oxygen.
Orthostatic	Drop in systolic blood pressure; hypotension > 10 mm Hg with change of position from supine to sitting or sitting to standing

BOX 5-11 Instructions for the Borg Rating of Perceived Exertion (RPE) Scale

During the work we want you to rate your perception of exertion (i.e., how heavy and strenuous the exercise feels to you and how tired you are). The perception of exertion is mainly felt as strain and fatigue in your muscles and as breathlessness, or aches in the chest. All work requires some effort, even if this is only minimal. This is true also if you only move a little (e.g., walking slowly).

Use this scale from 6 to 20, with 6 meaning "no exertion at all" and 20 meaning "maximal exertion."

- 6: "No exertion at all," means that you don't feel any exertion whatsoever (e.g., no muscle fatigue, no breathlessness, or difficulties breathing).
- 9: "Very light" exertion, such as taking a shorter walk at your own pace.
- A "Somewhat hard" work, but it still feels all right to continue.
- 15: It is "hard" and tiring, but continuing isn't terribly difficult.
- 17: "Very hard." This is very strenuous work. You can still go on, but you really have to push yourself and you are very tired.
- 19: An "extremely" strenuous level. For most people, this is the most strenuous work that they have ever experienced. Try to appraise your feeling of exertion and fatigue as spontaneously and as honestly as possible, without thinking about what the actual physical load is. Try not to underestimate and overestimate your exertion. It's your own feeling of effort and exertion that is important, not how this compares with that of other people. Look at the scale and the expressions and then give a number. Use any number you like on the scale, not just one of those with an explanation behind it.

Common chronic disorders of the lungs for which pulmonary rehabilitation is typically prescribed include chronic obstructive pulmonary disease (COPD) and asthma. COPD is characterized by damage to the alveolar wall and inflammation of the conducting airways and includes emphysema, peripheral airway disease, and chronic bronchitis. COPD has been diagnosed in more than 15 million Americans.

Emphysema is a condition in which the alveoli become enlarged or ruptured, usually because of a restriction during expiration or a decrease in the elasticity of the lungs. Chronic emphysema is most prevalent in men between the ages of 45 and 65 years who have a history of chronic bronchitis, smoking, working in areas with high levels of air pollution, or exposure to cold damp environments. Persons with chronic bronchitis experience shortness of breath (dyspnea) on exertion and, as the disease progresses, dyspnea occurs at rest.

Inflammation, fibrosis (thickening of the connective tissue), and narrowing of the terminal airways of the lungs are the physiologic changes that occur with peripheral airway disease. Smoking and other environmental pollutants irritate the airways, leading to the development of abnormal terminal airways. Coughing and spitting up mucus from the lungs are common clinical manifestations of this disorder. The disease process may never progress beyond this initial phase or it may evolve into emphysema and full-blown COPD.

Chronic bronchitis is diagnosed after a 2-year period of repeated episodes, greater than 3 months in length, of mucus-producing cough of unknown origin. A direct relationship exists between the development of chronic bronchitis and a history of cigarette smoking. Clinical manifestations of the disease increase as the package-year history increases. Pack-year history is calculated by multiplying the number of packs of cigarettes consumed per day by the number of years of smoking. Harriet began smoking at the age of 20. She is 64 years old now. Therefore, her pack-year history is $64 - 20 = 44 \times 1$ pack/day/year = 44 package years. As with other forms of COPD, the onset of physical disability is typically gradual, with dyspnea on exertion representing the initial phases of disability and devolving to shortness of breath at rest.

Asthma is characterized by irritability of the bronchotracheal tree and is typically episodic in its onset. Persons suffering from asthma experience wheezing and shortness of breath that may resolve spontaneously or may necessitate the use of medication for calming the airway. Those with asthma may be free of symptoms for periods of time between the episodes of wheezing and dyspnea. Some individuals appear to have a genetic predisposition to asthma. Allergenic causes of asthma may include pollens and respiratory irritants such as perfume, dust, pollen, and cleaning agents. Bronchospasms occurring with exposure to cold air or induced by exercise are sometimes the first clinical manifestations of asthma. Irritation of the airway leads to a narrowing of air passages and interferes with ventilation of the alveolar sacs. If the obstruction of the airway is significant enough, a reduction in oxygen levels in the bloodstream will result in hypoxemia. If left untreated, a severe asthmatic episode may result in death.

Pulmonary Rehabilitation

DYSPNEA CONTROL POSTURES

Adopting certain postures can reduce breathlessness. In a seated position, the patient bends forward slightly at the waist while supporting the upper body by leaning the forearms on the table or thighs. In a standing position, relief may be obtained by leaning forward and propping oneself on a counter or shopping cart.

Pursed-Lip Breathing

Pursed-lip breathing (PLB) is thought to prevent tightness in the airway by providing resistance to expiration. This technique has been shown to increase use of the diaphragm and decrease accessory muscle recruitment. Persons with COPD sometimes instinctively adopt this technique, whereas others may need to be taught it. Instructions for PLB are as follows:

1. Purse the lips as if to whistle.
2. Slowly exhale through pursed lips. Some resistance should be felt.
3. Inhale deeply through the nose.
4. It should take twice as long to exhale as it does to inhale.

Diaphragmatic Breathing

Another breathing pattern, which calls for increased use of the diaphragm to improve chest volume, is diaphragmatic breathing. Many persons learn this technique by placing a small paperback novel on the abdomen just below the xiphoid process (base of the sternum or breastbone). The novel provides a visual cue for diaphragmatic movement. The patient lies supine and is instructed to inhale slowly and make the book rise. Exhalation through pursed lips should cause the book to fall.

Relaxation

Progressive muscle relaxation in conjunction with breathing exercises can be effective in decreasing anxiety and controlling shortness of breath. One technique involves tensing muscle groups while slowly inhaling and then relaxing the muscle groups when exhaling twice as slowly through pursed lips. It is helpful to teach the patient a sequence of muscle groups to tense and relax. One common sequence involves tensing and relaxing first the face; followed by the face and the neck; then the face, neck, and shoulders; and so on, down the body to the toes. A calm, quiet, and comfortable environment is important for the novice in learning any relaxation technique. Biofeedback in conjunction with relaxation therapy promotes a more timely mastery of relaxation skills.

Other Treatments and Considerations

Physical therapists are generally called on to instruct the patient in chest expansion exercises, a series of exercises intended to increase the flexibility of the chest. Percussion and postural drainage use gravity and gentle drumming on the patient's back to loosen secretions and help drain the secretions from the lungs. By isometrically contracting his or her arms and hands while they are placed on the patient's thorax, the therapist may transmit vibration to the patient. Vibration is performed during the expiratory phase of breathing and helps loosen secretions. Percussion and postural drainage may be contraindicated in acutely ill patients and those who are medically unstable.

Humidity, pollution, extremes of temperature, and stagnant air have deleterious effects on persons with respiratory ailments. The therapist and patient should take these factors into consideration when planning activities.

Occupational Therapy Intervention

- Progression and energy costs
- Energy conservation
- Lifestyle modification
- Patient and family education

TABLE 5-27 Cardiovascular Response to Activity

Parameter	Response	
	Appropriate	Inappropriate
Heart rate (HR)	Increases with activity, to no more than 20 beats/min above resting heart rate	HR more than beats/min above resting heart rate (RHR); with activity, RHR ≥ 120 beats/min, HR drops or does not rise with activity
Blood pressure (BP)	Systolic blood pressure (SBP) rises with activity	SBP ≥ 220 mm Hg; postural hypotension (10-20 mm Hg drop in SBP); decrease in SBP with activity
Signs and symptoms	Absence of adverse symptoms	Excessive shortness of breath; angina; nausea and vomiting; excessive sweating; extreme fatigue (RPE ≥ 15); cerebral symptoms

RPE, Rate of perceived exertion.

TABLE 5-28 Basal Metabolic Equivalent Table of Self-Care and Homemaking Tasks

MET Level	Activities of Daily Living	Instrumental Activities of Daily Living, Work, Play, and Leisure
1-2	Eating, seated; transfers, bed to chair; washing face and hands; brushing hair; walking 1 mph	Hand sewing; machine sewing; sweeping floors; driving automatic car, drawing, knitting
2-3	Seated sponge bath; standing sponge bath; dressing and undressing; seated warm shower; walk 2-3 mph; wheelchair propulsion 1.2 mph	Dusting; kneading dough; hand washing small items; using electric vacuum; preparing a meal; washing dishes; golf
3-4	Standing shower, warm; bowel movement on toilet; climbing stairs at 24 ft/min	Making a bed; sweeping, mopping, gardening
4-5	Hot shower; bowel movement on bedpan; sexual intercourse	Changing bed linens; garden, rake, weed; rollerskate; swim 20 yards/min
5-6	Sexual intercourse; walking up stairs at 30 feet/min	Biking 10 mph on level ground
6-7	Walk with braces and crutches	Swim breaststroke; ski, play basketball, walk 5 mph, shovel snow, spade soil

Oncology

TABLE 5-29 Cancer Staging: TNM Definitions

Stage	Primary Tumor (T)	Nodal Involvement (N)	Distant Metastasis (M)
I	Tumor ≤ 5 cm in size; no invasion of adjacent tissues	No regional positive nodes	No (known) distant metastasis
II	Tumor > 5 cm in size; no invasion of adjacent tissues	No regional positive nodes	No (known) distant metastasis
III	Tumor outside organ in fat and surrounding soft tissues; tumor ≤5 cm in size; no invasion of adjacent tissues, or tumor > 5 cm in size; no invasion of adjacent tissues	No regional positive nodes Positive regional nodes	No (known) distant metastasis No (known) distant metastasis
IV	Tumor outside organ in fat and surrounding soft tissues, or tumor invading adjacent organs; tumor ≤ 5 cm in size; no invasion of adjacent tissues Tumor ≤ 5 cm in size; no invasion of adjacent tissues; tumor outside organ in fat and surrounding soft tissues, or tumor invading adjacent organs	Positive regional nodes No regional positive nodes or positive regional nodes	No (known) distant metastasis Distant metastasis present

Adapted from Norton JA, Le HN: Adrenal tumors. In DeVita VT Jr, Hellman S, Rosenberg SA (eds): *Cancer: Principles and practice of oncology,* 6th ed. Philadelphia, Lippincott Williams & Wilkins, 2001, pp 1770.

TABLE 5-30 Areas of OT Assessment and Intervention

Cancer Involvement (Body Structure/ Body Function)	Impairment	Activity Restriction	Participation Issues (Personal and Environmental Factors)
Brain	Motor	Mobility	Access
			Architectural barriers
			Adaptation
	Sensory	Safety/pain	Safety: need for supervision or a helper
			Pain: intolerance of participation in activities that exacerbate pain to level of intolerance
			Pain medicine: blurring senses, inability to drive or operate heavy machinery
	Cognitive	Planning	Inability to lead
		Sequencing	Lack of ability to plan or implement change
		Memory	
		Insight	
	Neurobehavioral	Safety	Social inappropriateness/stigma
	Visual impairment: hemianopsia, neglect, low vision, cortical blindness, loss of spatial relations perception.	Interference with ADLs/self-care and instrumental activities	Loss of occupational roles: work roles, family roles, ability to participate in leisure of sport activities
	Motor planning	Speaking	Inability to be independently involved in daily occupations
	Communication	Reading	Loss of major change in socialization and sharing ideas
		Writing	Severity of participation restriction dependent on individual interests and roles
Bone	Loss of motion	ADLs (basic and instrumental)	Ability to dress, bathe, toilet in context
	Pain		Need for adaptation of environment or presence of a caregiver
	Impaired mobility		Decreased ability to get around
	Risk of re-injury of affected part		Possible effect on employment
			Severity of participation restriction dependent on individual interests and roles

Breast	Loss of motion Pain Impaired mobility Risk of re-injury of affected part	ADLs (basic and instrumental) Shoulder mobility restrictions: sports, etc.	Temporary or long-term disruption in ability to do house-work, job, leisure activities Risk of injury because of lymphatic compromise; impact on sexuality
Lung	Shoulder mobility impairment (Pancoast tumor; post-thoracotomy) Impaired respiratory status Fatigue	ADLs (basic and instrumental) Shoulder mobility restrictions: sports, etc. Respiratory intolerance	Mobility issues respiratory tolerance and distance navigated Temporary or long-term disruption in ability to do house-work, job, leisure activities Risk of injury because of respiratory compromise Need for oxygen or nebulizing equipment
Colon	Change in way that bowels are managed (toileting-colostomy) Change in way body is washed (stomal issues) Chemoneuropathy impairment potential Fatigue	ADLs (basic and instrumental) Fatigue Social stigma of stoma (odor, bag ruptures, etc.) Fine motor impairment related to chemotherapy	Socially stigmatizing in community relationships
Prostate	Urinary incontinence Inability to perform sexually	ADLs (basic and instrumental)	Loss of sense of self as sexual being Stigma associate with incontinence
Head and neck	Inability to swallow/eat Loss of voice Neck and shoulder decrease in range of motion; loss of scapular stability	ADLs (feeding and eating; swallowing) Respiratory: management of oral secretions Bimanual overhead mobility activities Intimacy issues	Socially stigmatizing in community relationships Need to change contributory habits (smoking)

Special Needs of the Older Adult

Functional limitations caused by chronic conditions increase with age. More than one third of persons 65 years of age and older identify a chronic condition that imposes some limitation on everyday living, but only 10% report that the limitation affects a major activity. The four most frequently reported medical conditions in later life are arthritis, heart disease, hearing impairments, and orthopedic impairments. Of the old-old, age 75 years and older, 75% identify one disability; more than 50% identify two or more disabling conditions. Old-old adults have twice as many problems with ADLs as the young-old (65 to 74 years) adults. Of the old-old, 40% also have problems with IADLs. Despite chronic medical conditions, older adults are generally able to adapt and maintain function until very late in life.

Changes in Sensory Structures and Function

- Vision: Central field and peripheral field
- Treatment: Magnification, lighting, contrast, and organization
- Hearing: Presbycusis (gradual progressive loss)

Changes in Mental Structures and Function

- Sleep patterns
- Cognition
- Loss of memory
- Pathologic mental conditions
- Alcohol abuse
- Depression
- Suicide
- Anxiety disorders

Changes in Musculoskeletal Structures and Function

- Osteopenia
- Osteoporosis
- Osteoarthritis
- Muscle atrophy

Changes in Cardiovascular, Immunologic, and Respiratory Systems

- Blood pressure
- Heart rate
- Arteriosclerosis
- Atherosclerosis
- Immunologic function

Changes in Activities of Daily Living

- Incontinence
- Weight loss
- Poor dentition
- Swallowing
- Feeding
- Meal preparation
- Grocery shopping
- Functional mobility
- Falls
- Assistive devices for mobility
- Personal hygiene
- Sexual activity

Changes in Instrumental Activities of Daily Living

- Caring for others
- Community mobility
- Safety and emergency maintenance
- Rest and sleep
- Work
- Leisure
- Social participation
- Coping
- Caregiving
- Aging in place
- Wellness and aging

HIV Infection and AIDS

OTs may see a diverse population of people with AIDS, with numerous occupational deficits. Many physical and psychosocial factors indicate the need for an OT. Signs experienced by people with HIV and AIDS include, but are not limited to, the following:

- Fatigue and shortness of breath
- Impairment of the central nervous system (CNS)
- Impairment of the peripheral nervous system
- Visual deficits
- Sensory deficits (including painful neuropathies)
- Cardiac problems
- Muscle atrophy
- Altered ability to cope with and adapt to the changes that illness creates
- Depression
- Anxiety
- Guilt
- Anger
- Preoccupation with illness versus wellness

Pizzi Assessment of Productive Living for Adults with HIV Infection and AIDS (PAPL)

Demographics

Name_____Age_____

Sex_____Lives with (relationship)_____

Identified caregiver_____

Race _____Culture_____Religion_____

Practicing?_____How does spirituality play a role in your life, if

any?_____

Primary occupational roles:

_____

Primary diagnosis:

_____

Secondary diagnosis:

_____

Stage of HIV_____

Past Medical History:

_____

Medications:

_____

Activities of Daily Living (use ADL performance assessment)

Are you doing these now?

_____

Do you perform homemaking tasks?

_____

(For areas of difficulty) Would you like to be able to do these again like you did

before?_____ Which ones? _____

Work

Job _____When last worked_____

Describe type of activity_____

Work environment _____

If not working, would you like to be able to?_____

FIGURE 5-46 Pizzi Assessment of Productive Living for Adults with HIV Infection
and AIDS (PAPL). LTG, Long-term goals; STG, short-term goals. (Courtesy Michael
Pizzi 1991.)

Continued

Do you miss being productive?_____

Types of activity engaged in_____

If not, would you like to?_____Which ones?_____

Would you like to try other things as well?_____

Is it important to be independent in daily living activities?_____

Play/Leisure (interests and current participation)_____

_____

Sleep issues (habits, patterns)_____

Physical Function

Active and passive range of motion:

Strength:

Sensation:

Coordination (gross and fine motor or dexterity):

Visual-perceptual:

Hearing:

Balance (sit and stand):

Ambulation, transfers, and mobility:

Activity tolerance/endurance:

Physical pain:

Location:

_____

Does it interfere with doing important activities?_____

Sexual function:

Cognition

(Attention span, problem solving, memory, orientation, judgment, reasoning, decision making, safety awareness)

Time Organization

Former daily routine (before diagnosis)

FIGURE 5-46, cont'd

Has this changed since diagnosis?_____

If so, how? _____

Are there certain times of day that are better for you to carry out daily tasks?

_____

Do you consider yourself regimented in organizing time and activity or pretty

flexible? _____

What would you change, if anything, in how your day is set up?

_____

Body image and self-image

In the last 6 months, has there been a recent change in your physical body and how it

looks?_____How do you feel about this?_____

_____

Social environment (Describe support available and utilized by patient)

Physical environment (Describe environments where patient performs daily tasks and

level of support or impediment for function)

Stressors

What are some things, people, or situations that are/were stressful?_____

_____

What are some current ways you manage stress?_____

_____

Situational Coping

How do you feel you are dealing with:

a) your diagnosis

_____

_____

b) changes in the ability to do things important to you?

_____

_____

c) other psychosocial observations

_____

_____

FIGURE 5-46, cont'd

Continued

Occupational Questions

What do you feel to be important to you right now?

_____

Do you feel you can do things important to you now? In the future?

_____

Do you deal well with change?

_____

What are your hopes, dreams, aspirations? What are some of your goals?

_____

Have these changed since you were diagnosed? How?

_____

Do you feel in control of your life at this time?

_____

What do you wish to accomplish with the rest of your life?

_____

Plan:

STG:

LTG:

Frequency:

Duration:

Therapist:

FIGURE 5-46, cont'd

Polytrauma and Occupational Therapy

The term _polytrauma_ is now consistently used by U.S. military medical personnel and the Veterans Administration (VA) to describe the multiple, extreme, and often totally incapacitating complex traumatic injuries that service members suffer in the aftermath of war.

One of the most common causes of polytrauma is from exposure to a blast, such as that from an improvised explosive device (IED) or a rocket-propelled grenade (RPG).

- Primary blast injury is the result of exposure to the overpressurization wave or complex pressure wave that is generated by the blast itself. This blast overpressurization wave travels at a high velocity and is affected by the surrounding environment; for example, the effects of the blast wave may be increased in a closed environment such as a vehicle. Air-filled organs such as the ear, lung, and gastrointestinal tract and organs surrounded by fluid-filled cavities such as the brain and spinal cord are especially susceptible to primary blast injury. The overpressurization wave dissipates quickly, causing the greatest risk of injury to those closest to the explosion.

- Secondary blast injury is the result of energized fragments flying through the air; these fragments may cause penetrating brain injury.
- Tertiary blast injury may occur when the individual is thrown from the blast into a solid object such as an adjacent wall or even a steering wheel. These types of injuries are associated with acceleration and deceleration forces and blunt force trauma to the brain similar to that observed following high-speed MVAs.

Finally, a quaternary blast injury can occur in the presence of severe blast-related trauma resulting from significant blood loss associated with traumatic amputations or even from inhalation of toxic gases resulting from the explosion.

TABLE 5-31   Overview of Explosive-Related Injuries

System	Injury or Condition
Auditory or vestibular	Tympanic membrane rupture, ossicular disruption, cochlear damage, foreign body, hearing loss, distorted hearing, tinnitus, ear ache, dizziness, sensitivity to noise
Eye, orbit, face	Perforated globe, foreign body, air embolism, fractures
Respiratory	Blast lung, hemothorax, pneumothorax, pulmonary contusion and hemorrhage, arteriovenous fistulas (source of air embolism), airway epithelial damage, aspiration pneumonitis, sepsis
Digestive	Bowel perforation, hemorrhage, ruptured liver or spleen, sepsis, mesenteric ischemia from air embolism, sepsis, peritoneal irritation, rectal bleeding
Circulatory	Cardiac contusion, myocardial infarction from air embolism, shock, vasovagal hypotension, peripheral vascular injury, air embolism–induced injury
CNS	Concussion, closed and open brain injury, petechial hemorrhage, edema, stroke, small blood vessel rupture, spinal cord injury, air embolism-induced injury, hypoxia or anoxia, diffuse axonal injury
Renal	Renal contusion, laceration, acute renal failure due to rhabdomyolysis, hypotension, and hypovolemia
Extremity injury	Traumatic amputation, fractures, crush injuries, compartment syndrome, burns, cuts, lacerations, infections, acute arterial occlusion, air embolism-induced injury
Soft tissue	Crush injuries, burns, infections, slow healing wounds
Emotional or psychological	Acute stress reactions, PTSD, survivor guilt, postconcussive syndrome, depression, generalized anxiety disorder
Pain	Acute pain from wounds, crush injuries, or traumatic amputation; chronic pain syndromes

From Centers for Disease Control and Prevention (CDC): *Explosions and blast injuries: A primer for clinicians,* 2006 (http://www.bt.cdc.gov/masscasualties/explosions.asp).

A polytrauma transitional rehabilitation program (PTRP) provides comprehensive, postacute cognitive retraining and community reentry rehabilitation to TBI patients who have progressed beyond the needs of basic rehabilitation interventions. The goals of this program are to integrate clients back into the community, assist them with independent living, and help them return to their life roles. Not all clients who enter the PTRP program have been through the PRC; many are direct referrals from other VA facilities, from a polytrauma network site (PNS), and from outside private facilities or military treatment facilities. Because these clients have already achieved the goal of basic inpatient rehabilitation—that is, independence in ADLs and basic functional mobility—the focus while involved with the PTRP is on the higher level skills needed to return to the community. There is more of a cognitive retraining focus, with an emphasis on group work and community. Most clients reside within the PTRP facility, but some have already transitioned back to the community and come to the facility for the day program.

There has been a significant increase in the incidence of mild traumatic brain injury (mTBI) in services members as a result of serving in the Operation Enduring Freedom in Afghanistan and Operation Iraqi Freedom (OIF/OEF) conflict. There is no standard, agreed-on definition of mTBI. The U.S. Department of Veterans Affairs uses this definition of mTBI in all of its TBI screening evaluations: "A patient with mild traumatic brain injury is a person who has had a traumatically induced physiologic disruption of brain function as manifested by at least one of the following."

1. Any period of loss of consciousness
2. Any loss of memory for events immediately before or after the accident
3. Any alteration in mental state at the time of the accident (e.g., feeling dazed, disoriented, or confused)
4. Focal neurologic deficit(s) that may or may not be transient but where the severity of the injury does not exceed the following:
   a. Loss of consciousness of approximately 30 minutes or less
   b. After 30 minutes, an initial Glasgow Coma Scale (GCS) of 13 to 15
   c. Post-traumatic amnesia (PTA) not longer than 24 hours

Common symptoms of mTBI are headache, dizziness, nausea and vomiting, sleep disturbances, sensitivity to light, sensitivity to noise, slowed processing, memory difficulties, irritability, depression, and visual changes. An individual may experience symptoms at the time of the event or weeks after the mTBI. Most of those who sustain mTBI experience a resolution of symptoms within 3 months. However, 15% to 30% of individuals experience ongoing symptoms and may develop postconcussive syndrome. Postconcussive syndrome is when these symptoms or clusters of symptoms persist for more than 3 months.

Postconcussive syndrome can affect outcomes at any stage of polytrauma rehabilitation. Sometimes, those with postconcussive syndrome do not express themselves until many of the life-threatening injuries are stabilized. While in the acute phase of rehabilitation, the symptoms may affect function, but the focus may be more on the acute injury, not the persistent postconcussive symptoms. While in the postacute phase, postconcussive symptoms are identified during higher level functional activities. Patients can also be treated for post-traumatic stress disorder (PTSD) when mTBI and postconcussive symptoms are recognized.

Clients who experience multiple blast exposures are at higher risk of more complicated mTBIs. This, in conjunction with exposure to stressful environments, increases the risk of mTBI and acute stress reaction (ASR) or PTSD. This is true for mTBIs sustained in MVAs in the private sector as well. The stressful environment, multiple exposures, and ASR-PTSD can have a significant impact on the natural recovery from an mTBI.

The symptoms of acute stress reaction, depression, and PTSD are similar to those of mTBI postconcussive syndrome. This can include memory and concentration difficulties, sleep problems, impaired attention, irritability, and headache.

Bibliography

Unless otherwise noted, material is this field guide is derived from Pendleton HM, Schultz-Krohn W: *Pedretti's Occupational Therapy: Practice Skills for Physical Dysfunction,* ed 7, St. Louis, 2012, Elsevier, Inc.

Carter R, Lubinsky J, Domholdt E: *Rehabilitation Research: Principles and Applications,* ed 4, St. Louis, 2011, Elsevier, Inc.

Case-Smith J, O'Brien JC: *Occupational Therapy for Children,* ed 6, St. Louis, 2010, Elsevier, Inc.

Cook AM, Polgar JM: *Cook & Hussey's Assistive Technologies: Principles and Practice,* ed 3, St. Louis, 2008, Elsevier, Inc.

DePoy E, Gitlin LN: *Introduction to Research: Understanding and Applying Multiple Strategies,* ed 4, St. Louis, 2011, Elsevier, Inc.

Gillen G: *Cognitive and Perceptual Rehabilitation: Optimizing Function,* ed 1, St. Louis, 2009, Elsevier, Inc.

Gillen G: *Stroke Rehabilitation: A Function-Based Approach,* ed 3, St. Louis, 2011, Elsevier, Inc.

Ikiugu MN: *Psychosocial Conceptual Practice Models in Occupational Therapy: Building Adaptive Capability,* ed 1, St. Louis, 2007, Elsevier, Inc.

Quinn L, Gordon J: *Documentation for Rehabilitation: A Guide for Clinical Decision Making,* ed 2, St. Louis, 2010, Elsevier, Inc.

Index